Slow
Sex

Slow Sex

The Art and Craft of the Female Orgasm

NICOLE DAEDONE

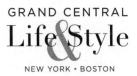

GRAND CENTRAL
Life & Style
NEW YORK · BOSTON

This book is not intended as a substitute for medical advice of physicians. The reader should regularly consult a physician in all matters relating to his or her health, and particularly in respect of any symptoms that may require diagnosis or medical attention.

Copyright © 2011 by IP Media, Inc.

Grand Central Life & Style
Hachette Book Group
237 Park Avenue
New York, NY 10017

Grand Central Life & Style is an imprint of Grand Central Publishing. The Grand Central Life & Style name and logo are trademarks of Hachette Book Group, Inc.

Printed in the United States of America

ISBN 978-0-446-56719-0

This book is dedicated to the orgasm.
May each of us find ours now.

Contents

Introduction

When I first tell people I make my living teaching the art of Slow Sex, I get to watch as an entire weather system crosses their faces in a matter of about five seconds. First I see surprise, then curiosity, then embarrassment about their curiosity, then fear that I can see their embarrassment, then—finally—the courage to proceed.

"What...exactly...do you mean by Slow Sex?" they venture, so carefully you'd think they were carrying a piece of fine china across a tightrope.

Ah, sex. As soon as you say the word, we all get a little wobbly. We're just so used to keeping it in private that when I come along and start talking about it publicly, everyone is caught a little off guard.

"I teach a practice called Orgasmic Meditation," I say as calmly as possible. "It's a way that any man can bring out the orgasm in any woman, in just fifteen minutes."

You can imagine the response: surprise, then curiosity, then embarrassment...you know the drill. It's not like I'm lying—even though it's called Slow Sex, Orgasmic Meditation or OM does show men how to make any woman orgasmic in just fifteen minutes—but it's not as big a deal as it sounds. Yes, it can be life changing. Yes, it turns everything we've ever learned about sex on its head. But what I teach people when I teach them OM is really no different from what my Uncle Bob taught me one summer afternoon when I was twelve years old. That was the day he taught me how to really, truly taste a tomato.

Uncle Bob and the Tomato

I grew up in suburban Los Gatos, California, hardly a hub of modern agriculture. But it was the 1970s, and because all of the old structures seemed to be crumbling—and probably in part because everyone wanted to start growing their own marijuana—lots of suburbanites convinced themselves they were farmers. Mrs. Calder put a "Love Your Mother" bumper sticker on her Lincoln Town Car. My friend Shea's family made plans to buy a dome house in Grass Valley. And in the backyards of our cul-de-sac, Mrs. Farrier grew corn, Mr. Slocum grew strawberries, and my uncle Bob—who always set an example because he worked for *Rolling Stone* magazine and had the longest beard—grew potatoes, beans, snap peas, and sweet, glorious tomatoes.

I remember the first basket of heirloom tomatoes that my overall-wearing uncle presented to my mother in our gold-and-avocado-colored kitchen.

"Jesus, Bob, they look deformed. Are we really supposed to eat them?"

Bob, not to be insulted, picked up one of the deformed tomatoes and took a bite out of it, as if it were an apple. This I had never seen in my decade-plus on this planet. Tomatoes were to be sliced and carefully arranged on a plate, not bitten into haphazardly in the middle of the kitchen so that the juices dripped down your chin and into your very long beard.

Bob smiled broadly and offered the tomato to my mother.

My mother, not yet having succumbed to the seventies back-to-the-earth ethos, still using hair spray with fluorocarbons, wasn't sure what to make of it. She leaned hesitantly over the sink to protect her minidress, and took a delicate bite. When she looked up at my uncle, the expression on her face was pure bliss. In slow motion, she turned and handed me the tomato. I looked up at the two of them, a bit nervous. I felt the way I would later feel when someone handed me my first joint. What would happen to me if I ate this tomato?

But I bit in and I understood. Rich, earthy, dense. The taste of minerals. Where previous tomatoes had been porous, spongy, common—this tomato was pure saturation. It was as if the tomato itself had a built-in speed limit; it was not possible to eat it quickly and forget about it. There was a there there. This tomato took command. There was no mistaking it: this was a tomato!

My uncle asked me what I tasted.

I couldn't speak. I didn't want to break the spell.

"What do you taste?" he prodded, as if he were a blind man asking me what I saw. I wanted to sound very smart, to impress him. A difficult task when what you're describing is a tomato.

"It tastes . . . warm? And a little sour."

"Yes! Yes!" He gestured for more.

"It's kind of like when you lick a penny. It tastes like metal and you feel a sort of jolt."

"Yes!"

"But at the end, it makes your mouth water. It's sweet, but not candy sweet. Sweet the way skin smells. Soft."

My uncle was pleased. He put his hands on my shoulders and looked in my eyes as if this were it—as if at that very moment I was heading out on the vision quest of life, and he was offering me just one last piece of advice.

"Nic," he said, "the most important thing you will ever do in this life is to really taste a tomato."

I often think back about that day in the kitchen when I'm getting ready to teach Slow Sex to a new group of students. Students who are coming to my class because their sex lives seem mealy, unflavorful, and common. They have never tasted anything like an heirloom; they aren't even sure sex that is saturating, nourishing, and delicious beyond expectation actually exists. They think of sex the way I thought about tomatoes. I had been living a vacuum-sealed suburban life where everyone bought their tomatoes from the Shop 'n Save and nobody talked about the fact that they weren't delicious. Nobody really talked about the tomatoes at all. What was there to talk about? Tomatoes were tomatoes.

Then came Uncle Bob, and the revelation that there were tomatoes on this planet that were worth your time. Tomatoes that begged to be really *tasted*—that asked you to plug into them with all of your attention and all of your senses. Tomatoes that offered the richness of the earth and sky in return. My students are wary at first, just like I was. They have hesitation; they aren't sure whether to trust that better sex is available. So all I can do is give them a taste and let them see for themselves.

It's my job to help them make contact with the heirloom variety of sex, the best that sex has to offer. And then, to teach them how to taste every rich, nourishing moment. To show them how they, too, can be saturated by the nutrients available in their very own soil, how they can taste and be tasted. And how the kind of sex we've been settling for, just because it's what's available at the Shop 'n Save, is not the only option. Like my uncle's tomato, an heirloom variety is available—you just have to know where to go looking for it.

Several years after I first tasted the tomato, I had forgotten the lesson Uncle Bob taught me that day. I was twenty years old and thought I knew everything there was to know about everything. In truth, of course, I knew nothing about anything. But I did know that something wasn't going right in my life.

Outwardly all was well: I'd graduated magna cum laude and was already doing my master's work in a field I loved. I had the first paid teaching assistant position in my department and had been taken in by a prestigious mentor. I was living in one of the most sophisticated and interesting cities in the country—San Francisco—and I was in a "great relationship."

Like a good girl, I had built this perfect-looking life, and now I was supposed to—what? Enjoy it? If someone could have told me how to do that, I would have been in better shape. But as it was, I was bored as hell. I felt like I was withering on the vine. It's like I was eating and eating and eating, but I never felt full; this whole fantastic life I'd set up for myself was giving me nothing but an empty stomach. I knew something more had to be available—I could hear it calling me at night while I lay staring at the ceiling, wondering how my life could be over before it had even begun—but I didn't know where to find more vitality, more engagement, more of the everything I wanted.

Then a friend told me she was taking a course in sexuality. I was momentarily scandalized. Sexuality was something good girls like me didn't talk about!

Then I was curious. Then embarrassed at my curiosity. Then a little bit afraid, and then, a little bit courageous.

I signed up for the class with her, and that was the beginning of the rest of my life. If Uncle Bob had been there, he would have been smiling.

More Is Possible

As it turned out, the "me" who knew nothing about anything actually sensed something very important. Just one little thing. She sensed that, somehow, the place to look for help in relearning how to be touched by her own life was sex. You, too, know that intuitively. Otherwise you wouldn't be holding this book. Instead you'd have given up on sex, abandoned all hope of relationship satisfaction, and/or joined a monastery. But no: you're making the radical choice to move toward your sexuality rather than away from it. Because you know that it's in sex where all the real nourishment lies, and you're sick of empty calories.

It's been more than two decades since I took that first class. Now I make my living teaching sexuality to others—to men and women, younger and older, gay and straight, who are in the same boat I was in when I first took the leap into my sexuality and, as it turned out, my life. People who have that same intuition, that little voice that whispers something more has to be possible here. What I want to say to my twenty-year-old self—and to each of the students I see in class—is this: You are right! More is possible.

At the time, I wouldn't have imagined how much impact sex would have on my sense of fulfillment and happiness. Like lots of people, I saw sex as sort of a side dish to the main meal of my life. Though I'd always been a sexual person, I still considered my sexuality to be extracurricular. It was something I used for stress reduction, pleasure, escape, or at the best of times to feel close to someone. But if you'd told me then that sex would end up being the center of my life—that here, a couple of decades later, I'd be spending my time teaching people Slow Sex, that I would have founded OneTaste, a national organization devoted to the art and craft of the female orgasm—I would have thought you were nuts. I was there on a lark—to break the monotony of my life and to maybe learn how to have better orgasms in the process. I certainly didn't think I was going to discover the key to sustainable happiness.

But, as life would have it, that's exactly what happened. What I discovered in that class was that sexuality is not just a fringe activity, an exceptionally fun hobby. Instead I saw it for what it really is: a source of power, a well from which I could draw the energy I needed to discover who I was and how I wanted to live my life. And how I wanted to live my life was to enjoy it, for heaven's sake. To feel full and energized so I could live every moment of it to its absolute fullest potential. Sex turned out to be the entry point to the deep, nourishing joy that every part of me was crying out for, as well as the fuel that would get me there. Once I tasted this heirloom variety of sexuality, there was nothing else I wanted to cultivate in my life.

Everything you were hoping was possible in sex is possible. Sex can be so much more than we have come to believe. It can be a gateway to more connection, more vitality, and more sensation in all areas of our lives. All we have to do is explore it with the mind of a beginner. To leave behind the menu that's been handed down to us, with all of its rules and expectations, and feel our way. Offering you the sexuality practices in this book is my version of handing you the tomato. I will show you how to take that first bite, how to really taste it. The rest will take care of itself.

Why You Picked Up This Book

I always start my Slow Sex workshops by asking the students what brings them to be sitting in front of me, here in a sex class. Once they get past the embarrassment of being reminded that they are in fact sitting in front of me, in a sex class, their responses fall into one of four categories.

1. They've heard about Slow Sex, and they're just plain curious. Can any woman really have an orgasm, every time? Could all the hype be true?
2. As a man, they want a foolproof technique for pleasing any woman, anytime.
3. As a woman, they want to actually experience the pleasure they know they're supposed to be getting from sex, but can't seem to access.
4. They just want more from their sex lives than they are currently getting, and they have an intuition that Slow Sex may help.

The first group never leaves the workshop disappointed. Sex is maybe the most interesting subject on the planet, and we're about to talk about it—a lot. We're going to roll up our sleeves and really get into it ourselves, in a way few workshops dare.

Yes, I mean that pants will be coming off.

And that every woman in class is going to be revealed as mind-blowingly orgasmic.

In other words, the curious are going to get what they came for.

Now, don't get me wrong: the others are curious, too, but they tend to be on a more specific mission. The men desperately (more desperately than their partners can possibly imagine) want to be better at pleasing their women. On the surface level, they know that the more she's getting out of sex, the more often they'll have it. The deeper desire they have—which many of them aren't even aware of—is the desire to have sex with a woman who is truly turned on. They know that the more turned on their partner is, the better their own experience will be.

For their part, the women I see want to know how to receive the pleasure their men so desperately want to give them. They, too, want to be turned on beyond their wildest imagination—but they haven't been able to figure out how. Often the harder he tries, the less into it she is. Some women think it's that their partner is not sexy or talented enough; some fear that they, themselves, are blocked or frozen in some way. Regardless of the reason, these women are here because they're hoping Slow Sex will show them how to be the fully orgasmic beings they know—or at least hope—they really are.

And the last group—everybody who didn't fit into the first three—can be summarized in one sentence: they just want *more*. More sex, more sensation, more pleasure, more connection—more, pure and simple. It takes courage to admit you want more from your sex life. It can be taboo and embarrassing to say that we're not 100 percent satisfied with what we already have. If you don't believe me, try being a sex teacher for a day. It turns out to be a great conversation stopper at dinner parties. People who individually might voice their curiosity clam up pretty quick when they're in a group. Everyone at the table will nod politely as if saying, "That's nice for you, but me? I don't need it. Perrrrfectly happy over here, yep."

Afterward, of course, half the table will try to catch me on my way to the bathroom to talk my ear off about their sex lives. How they've never had an orgasm, how they want sex more or less frequently than their partner does, how they have no idea how a woman's apparatus is put together, or how they have no interest in sex at all anymore and want to know if I have any hope to offer.

These are all variations on the same themes I hear from my students, many of whom are on the verge of giving up on finding satisfying sex and deep intimacy by the time they find me. They've gone looking for answers before. Big promises, free giveaways, infomercials—nothing has hit the chord they're looking for. When I hear how hard they've been working—how much effort they've put into the battle to win over their own sexuality—it's hard to believe they didn't raise the white flag a long time ago.

And yet, they still come. They come for the same reason I walked into my first sexuality class. They have an intuition that there's something they need to address, something vital, something that has to do with life and happiness and satisfaction, something that can be found only if they are willing to slow down and really feel their sexuality. If they're willing to learn something new, take a new approach to sex. The men are not satisfied with the cultural myth that women will never enjoy sex as much as they do. The women are not willing to give in to the idea that sexual desire inevitably wanes with age and familiarity, and that they should just get used to the idea that sex with their partner will become less satisfying over time. If that's the case, they tell me, they want off this bus. They're not going to settle for less than deep connection and saturation, and they'll keep looking until they find the answer.

The answer that gives men a foolproof way to pleasure their woman every time. That translates "womanspeak" so they can understand it. That releases them from performance anxiety. That gives them permission to relax and enjoy sex, knowing they are getting it right.

The answer that shows women how to sink down and truly *feel* during sex, to bring the locus of their sexuality back into their own bodies where they can use it to get more turned on than they ever thought possible. That shows them how to use turn-on as an energy source rather than a drain. The answer that shows them how to let go of the expectation that their orgasm should look and sound like this or that. That truly gives them permission to enjoy the journey, rather than pushing them ever sooner to the finale.

The answer everyone is looking for is Slow Sex. Like the Slow Food movement, which turned the emphasis from fast-food convenience and cost-efficiency toward sustainable practices and eating for enjoyment, Slow Sex is a way to approach sex that emphasizes sustainability, connection, and nourishment. It deepens your relationship to your partner and your own body, so you can experience orgasm from the inside out. Like Slow Food, Slow Sex is a philosophy—a philosophy of stripping sex down to its most basic state, learning to feel it deeply in the body, and communicating our desires. But in the same way that you can't really understand Slow Food until you take the first bite, Slow Sex cannot be understood unless it is experienced. We primarily experience Slow Sex through the practice of Orgasmic Meditation—OM or OMing (pronounced "om-ing") for short. OMing itself is not sex—it's a simple, meditative practice where the man strokes the woman's genitals for fifteen minutes. But the skills we develop while OMing are nothing short of revolutionary when applied to traditional sex. So while the primary focus of this book, and Slow Sex in general, is the practice of OM, that's only the first step. The real experience of Slow Sex happens when you extend the philosophy—stripping down, feeling your sensations, and asking for what you want—into the realm of "regular" sex. So, later in the book, I will offer practices in how to apply these three principles of Slow Sex to intercourse, oral sex, and more.

In Orgasmic Meditation we learn to shift our focus from thinking to feeling, from a goal orientation to an experience orientation. This shift turns all our expectations about sex on their head, exchanging "faster" and "harder" for "slower" and "more connected." There is no longer any planned outcome to sex, no goal—not even climax—that is expected. Instead, Slow Sex teaches us how to feel and enjoy the orgasm we are having right now: to savor every stroke and every sensation along the way. As many students and Slow Sex coaching clients have already discovered, the results of this practice are much greater than the sum of their parts. Here's some of what you can expect:

Introduction

"I feel so much more confident knowing that I am giving my wife pleasure every time. OM is like the secret ingredient. The kind of sex we're having is the kind I had always been looking for."　　　　　　　　　　　　　　—Craig, 43

"I don't think I ever really felt sex before I started OMing. Now I can feel my sexual energy all the time, even after the OM is over."　　　　　　　　　　　　　　—Jen, 31

"Whereas before I only really felt aroused in my genitals, now my entire body is an erogenous zone."　　　　—Kurt, 52

"I have learned how to really let my sexuality come out and play. It's like I was holding back all this time and didn't even know it. Now I have permission to let it out and enjoy sex in a whole new way."　　　　　　　　　　　—Liz, 28

"Since we've been practicing Orgasmic Meditation, my girlfriend is so much more turned on. I can't believe how different it is to have sex with a woman who is truly turned on."　　　　　　　　　　　　　　　　　　—Jon, 40

"I thought I wasn't attracted to my husband anymore, but OMing has changed everything. The more we OM, the more I want to have sex."　　　　　　　—Suzanne, 41

What OM teaches is actually transferable into *all* of our relationships—even into life in general. All we have to do is open our lens beyond the conventional understanding of sex and orgasm—especially when it comes to *her* experience. Though traditionally the centerpiece of sex has been

13

the male orgasm, Slow Sex turns our attention toward the female orgasm. And once you enter her world, nothing will ever be the same again.

Every Woman Is Orgasmic...No, Seriously

They say we all have our blind spots, but when it comes to sex, we all have the same one. Ask a hundred people what it takes for a man to have an orgasm, and hands will shoot up all over the room. Men and women both know the male equipment like the back of their hands, and for the most part, one size fits all. But ask that same group of people for the formula that will make a *woman* orgasmic, and the show of hands will be sparse at best. Everybody knows how to get him off, but she's more...complicated. Women themselves often see their own sexuality as, if you will, a black box. Thanks to cultural conditioning that says a woman's parts are best kept in the dark, many women have a hard time feeling connected to their genitals—and thus, their own orgasm.

Which, as it turns out, is very different from a man's.

So when we compare her orgasm to his (which we do) and hold his orgasm as the model she should be striving for (which we do), then her orgasm can look like a problem child who sometimes refuses to come to the party. Fingers get pointed at both men and women. If he "can't get his woman off," then he's not sexy enough, not "giving" enough, or worse—he's (insert stage whisper) *not especially talented.* For the untalented man, there are bookshelves overflowing with guides promising to unlock the mysteries of her pleasure. For her part, if she can't come every time, then she's "frigid," stressed out, doesn't like sex, and/or doesn't know how to relax. Again, there are books, toys, sensitizing lubricants, and sexy lingerie that promise to fix this major problem that has befallen her. (Or more accurately, that she has brought onto herself by not being sexual/relaxed/comfortable enough to just come, already!) It's because of this cultural conundrum that I headline the practice of Slow Sex with this radical statement:

I have never met a woman who is not, right now, at this moment, orgasmic.

Yes, I mean *you.*

Yes, I mean *your* wife/girlfriend/lover.

Every woman, like every person, is orgasmic at every moment. Once you understand this, you're well on your way to understanding Slow Sex.

That said, it usually takes a little while for my students to adjust to this new world order. The puzzlement they experience stems from a misunderstanding of the word "orgasmic." We have been defining the term "orgasm" as the traditional definition of *male* orgasm: climax. Contrary to what we learned in sex education (and as teenagers rolling around on the living room floor desperately hoping our parents didn't walk in) climax is not synonymous with orgasm. *Orgasm is the body's ability to receive and respond to pleasure.* Pure and simple. Climax is often a *part* of orgasm, but it is not the sum total. Make this distinction, and you change the whole game.

You discover that women are just as orgasmic as men— maybe even more so.

You discover that women want sex as much as men do—just not the sex that's usually on the menu.

You start to realize that climax is like reading just the

last line of a book—you can do it, sure, but you'll miss out on the whole story.

Make this discovery, and suddenly all of our expectations about sex, orgasm, women and men, relationships, and life get reset. Now, isn't it about time?

About This Book

This book is an introduction to the philosophy of Slow Sex and the practice of Orgasmic Meditation. It's modeled on my Slow Sex workshops and is meant as a beginner's guide—an instruction manual that will allow you to begin practicing the principles of Slow Sex right away (or by the end of chapter 3, at any rate). I have set it up in much the same way you would learn the content if you were with me in class. First, we'll talk about what Slow Sex is and why you'd want to practice it in the first place. Then I'll walk you step by step through the practice of Orgasmic Meditation, including our "Ten Day Starter Program," which will help you and your partner build a sustainable—and don't forget enjoyable—practice. Once we've got you OMing, I'll tell you all sorts of other secrets: what OM teaches us about women, men, and sex, right up to and including instructions for how to have a four-month orgasm. (Try not to skip ahead. Just try.)

In addition to the OM practice, I've included a variety of experiential exercises guaranteed to bring the Slow Sex revolution right to the comfort of your very own home. The core practice of OM and most of the other sexuality practices in the book require a partner. If you don't currently have a partner or friend-with-benefits to practice with, don't worry; there's still a lot to learn. The ultimate outcome of OM is to return the center of our sexual universe to our very own bodies. We've come to believe that our sexuality depends upon the right *external* circumstances—a partner who wants to have sex with us, say, or a body we're willing to let see the light of day. But in reality, sexuality arises from the inside out. So the work I'm teaching in this book begins with you. My OM workshops are open to individual practitioners as well as couples, and there is wisdom here for those who ultimately take up the practice and for those who do not. So don't worry if you don't have a partner right now: either you will be intrigued enough by the end of the book to find one, or you can keep your focus—well, more focus—on reviving your own sexuality and the way you relate to your world.

Speaking of individual experience, please take this book at your own pace. Looking deeply at your own sexuality isn't always easy. We have so much negative conditioning around sex, it's really a wonder anyone decides to dive into Slow Sex at all. I remember when I first realized that sexuality was my vocation. I went to tell my mother that her only child, who'd been wandering for so long, had finally discovered her life's calling. She was thrilled to hear I'd landed on something—until she heard *what* I'd landed on. Mom practically crumpled into a heap on the floor when I told her it was sex. I had to poke at her with a finger to make sure she was still breathing. Of course I felt bad. Not so much because she was disappointed in me (which she clearly was) or because she was going to beat herself up for whatever mistakes she'd made that had led her only daughter to *this* (which she did—for a while), but because I saw, through her response, the way all of us feel about sexuality, to some degree or another. Sex was so bad that my mere participation in it had my mother trading in her minidress for a black shroud. I made a promise then and there that I would devote myself to making the place I was going—the world of sexuality—less painful for everyone, Mom included.

So don't worry if you start to get the heebie-jeebies as you read this book. (If so, feel free to jump to chapter 4, Trouble-shooting, where you'll discover that you're far from alone.) Freak-outs come with the territory. Take things slowly, and work within your right range. You may feel like you've found the practice you've been looking for your whole life, or you may think OM is completely insane. You may run to your computer to sign up for a Slow Sex teleclass or workshop,[1] or you may decide you will heretofore avoid San Francisco entirely and forever for fear of running into yours truly. You may read the whole book in one sitting, or you may put it down and come back to it in a week or a month or a year. Whatever your response, go with it. The process of recon-necting with your sexuality looks different for everyone. It happens only as fast as it is supposed to happen. My request is that you simply follow your own desire. Feel for the sweet spot. What do you want? If you want to keep reading, do. If you want to do the practices, do. If not, don't. Whatever you do, make sure you're doing it out of desire. It's the only com-pass you've been given in this world, and you *can* trust it. It may not lead you where you thought you were going, but it will never lead you astray.

Nicole Daedone
San Francisco, CA
May 2010

---

1. Hey, just in case: www.onetaste.us

Chapter One

The Art of Slow Sex

As I stand in front of my new students on the first day of a Slow Sex workshop, it's like I'm a captain at the prow of a ship on a foggy night. The mist that hangs in the air between me and the class is so thick I can hardly see their faces.

It's the mist of abject terror. Holy mother, they're in a *sex class*.

Through the fog they're sizing me up, checking me out. If they're in a sex class, then I must be the sex teacher. *So that's what a sex teacher looks like.* It's hard not to open my mouth and say something hot, raunchy, and shocking just to see how far they'll jump out of their seats.

Alas, when I open my mouth the first thing I start talking about is my grandma. Not as titillating as they're hoping for, I realize, but there's nothing I can do. Grandma is where it all begins.

I was an only child, raised by my mother and my grandma. Grandma was an amazing cook. She was an old world–style cook, an immigrant from the Ukraine who knew how to make a mean borscht. Cooking for her loved ones—and

I was at the top of that list—was her favorite thing to do. She was a force of nature both in and out of the kitchen, and I was half afraid of her, half in love with her. I would watch her move from stove to sink to refrigerator with the precision of a dancer, the fascination of watching her cook outweighing the consequences of getting in her way.

Then, when I was fifteen, Grandma had a heart attack. The whole family was on edge, waiting. When the diagnosis came, there was good news and bad news. The good news was that she would survive; the bad news was that the condition was degenerative, and her heart was deteriorating. They didn't know how long she would live.

I was in a Home Ec class at the time, and I was cooking up a storm. Since Grandma was always cooking for everyone else, I thought, I will bring her something we make in class to show her how much I love her. So one afternoon after she got home, I brought her a dish we'd prepared that day. I set it on the table with great fanfare, waiting expectantly for her to take her first bite and shower me with praise. What happened was not what I was looking for, to say the least. She took a bite, yes, but she spit it back out before she even chewed it. I was shocked and then asked her what was wrong.

"You killed this food with the recipe," she said, matter-of-factly, and got up to start dinner.

I was, of course, mortified. But more than that, I was confused. What did she mean, I'd killed the food with the recipe? I made this thing in *class*, lady. A class I'm getting an A in, thank you very much. The whole point was to follow the recipe. If you don't follow a recipe, I stewed, how are you supposed to know how to cook the freaking dish?

Once I regained control of my hormone-driven teenage

emotions, I entered the kitchen and asked her, as calmly as possible, how one learned to cook without a recipe. She turned her ancient gaze toward me. I remember she looked tired, but wise. After a long pause she said, with what sounded like resignation, "Okay. I will teach you."

And with that, I started learning what it meant to cook without a recipe. For my first lesson, she said, I would go to the Russian supermarket and buy her favorite cabbage cigarettes. She would stay home and make soup.

There were toilets to clean after that, and other household chores to be done in entirely different parts of the house. All this while she stood in the kitchen and cooked. I tried not to be irritated, but I've never been very good at trying not to be something I am. I huffed and puffed, taking great pains to stomp past the kitchen as often as possible so she could get a taste of what *I* was cooking. But if she sensed my annoyance, she never showed it—she just let me drag the vacuum cleaner up and down the hallway as noisily as I pleased and never said a thing.

A friend asked me if I wanted to go to the mall after school. "No," I said. "My grandma is teaching me how to cook."

"Cool," she said.

"Hrumpf," I replied.

But then one day I showed up, and as I headed for the vacuum closet, Grandma summoned me to the kitchen.

"Today," she said, "we will make pierogi."

Once my disbelief wore off, I started jumping up and down. She shot me a look that told me to check my enthusiasm and put on an apron. (How do old women communicate so much with just one sideways glance?) At the counter, she let me watch as she mixed the flour and eggs and water to make the dough. Then it was my turn. She turned the dough out onto the floury counter, and told me to knead it. I had barely made a turn of the dough before she was behind me, pinching my arm. "Feel that? That's what you're doing to the dough! How do you think it feels, being pinched like that?"

I looked at her like she was insane. How does the *dough* feel? But a few more corrective arm pinches and I was massaging that dough with the same care and attention you'd use to powder a baby's bottom. Soon, I announced I was done and the dough was ready to be rolled out.

"How do you know it's done?" Grandma asked.

It was a good question. How *did* I know it was done? I don't know. It just was—it was done. Grandma looked at me with an expression at once amused and relieved.

"You are ready now, Nicole," she said.

~

That one day in the kitchen changed my life. In Home Ec, we learned to cook by finding a recipe and following its instructions exactly. We were rewarded for this good behavior by getting a meal and a good grade. In my grandma's world, we were getting into relationship with the food. Feeling it. Getting to know it. Learning how it wanted to be cooked. I wasn't even allowed to put on the apron until I was in relationship with my grandma—until I knew what cigarettes she liked to smoke and how she wanted her toilet bowl cleaned. Now I was getting into relationship with the dough, discovering how it wanted to be kneaded.

My grandma was teaching me the most important lesson of cooking, but also of living: anything you really get into relationship with will reveal its secrets to you. All you have to do is stand in the kitchen with an open mind and heart, recognizing the honor of cooking food for your family. The recipe will come.

This is a lesson I have never forgotten. It was the lesson of learning the difference between cooking as a science and cooking as an art. In science, we know that you make a cake by mixing together sugar and flour and eggs. You start from a position of knowledge—from a well-tested recipe—and you follow its rules until you have a cake. But for Grandma, the process started with a question: how does this particular cake *want* to be put together? These approaches come from two entirely different worlds. The first is the world of science—the science of cooking, but also of living. You take these rules, you apply them, and assuming you do it all right, the result is pretty much guaranteed. The second is where you begin to move into the *art* of living. You don't know where you're going and the results aren't guaranteed. You can give every single thing you have and not achieve the outcome you were hoping for. But what you do achieve is the experience of intimate relationship. You open yourself, and the answers come through you. You find that you know things you never knew before. You discover that a masterpiece doesn't actually require you to master anything at all. It simply requires you to feel, to listen, and to trust yourself. That's art.

The Art of Sex

Anything you do can be approached as either science or art—including, perhaps most important, sex. The kind of sex we all wish we were enjoying all the time is the kind we have when we approach sex as an art form rather than a science. The kind of sex that asks us to be open and curious and to follow the experience where it wants to go, rather than forcing it to head in the direction we think it's "supposed" to go, the direction the recipe *says* it should go in.

And yet most of the time, we treat sex like a science. We develop very strong expectations, anticipating a replicable outcome every time we add water and mix. We believe that "good" sex means one thing—probably something like mutual orgasms and a feeling of intimate connection to our partner—and that if either of the above is missing, the sex is "unsatisfying" or "truly problematic" or, worse yet, simply "good enough." We ignore the reality, which is that sex itself is messy and inconsistent. It is a force of nature, like my grandma. It is a reflection of life, which means it includes hot and cold, fast and slow, good and bad. Sometimes we want it, other times we don't. Sometimes we feel close to our partner, other times we feel like they might be a serial killer, for all we know. Sometimes we think they're the best lover in the world, other times we wish that someone, at some point during their teen years, had taught them how to *kiss,* for crying out loud. Some of us can climax from one touch, whereas others go all night and never "get there." Some of us remember a time when sex *used* to be great, but we can't for the life of us remember how to get there again. This is the reality of sex. Sex is not a science; there is no recipe. No matter how many books you read or how many repetitive motions you make, the outcome is not guaranteed. And mere inconsistency is the best-case scenario. The worst-case scenario? You kill the sex with the recipe.

But we've never learned to cook without a recipe—in

the kitchen or the bedroom. So when things don't turn out the way we expect, we find ourselves trying harder. Rather than opening up and letting our sexuality tell us what it wants in that moment, we try harder to comply with the external recipe we've been given. Rather than listening for our own desire and following it whether it makes sense or not, we try ever harder to be the good little recipe-follower we were taught to be. Pretty soon we've kneaded the dough into a tough, unappetizing lump.

Let's take the example of orgasm. While men's orgasms are also an art form, I think we can all agree that they tend to have more of that consistent scientific quality to them than women's orgasms do. If you'll pardon me for being blunt, "penis" plus "naked woman" in more cases than not does in fact equal "ejaculation." But what, then, happens when the recipe doesn't lead to the desired outcome? When no matter how hard he tries, the recipe—ahem—no longer stands on its own?

And then you've got women's orgasm, which for most of us follows a path much more like *The Artist's Way* than the scientific method. When observed objectively, women's orgasm looks very different from men's orgasm, and it may or may not include a climax. So what happens when we're following the recipe for "good sex," and (per usual) it calls for "two climaxes," and two climaxes are not available?

What happens in either of these cases—and in so many more and different ways where the truth of "no recipe" is revealed—is that sex starts looking like a problem. Because we're human and we exist in a paradigm of wrong (more on this later), we are trigger-happy when it comes to identifying problems. We are always on the lookout for someone or something to blame. We think there's something wrong with us, or with our relationship, or with our partner. The artsy-ness of sex, its frustrating refusal to abide by the laws of mechanics, puts us into the difficult position of wondering why things aren't going the way they're "supposed" to be going. Each of us tends to respond in a different way.

Men approach the problem of sex like they're trying to fix a TV that's on the fritz. They scratch their heads and try to figure it out. They ask investigative questions, tinker with this and that, and when the screen is still blank, they'll either become frustrated or zone out altogether.

For women, on the other hand, the tendency is to try to make her sex—and especially her orgasm—*look* a particular way, the way it's "supposed" to look. We try to live up to the expectations set by Hollywood, and *Cosmo,* and our best friend, Katie (who seems to *always* be having amazing sex, all the freaking time, and who never really gets that *we don't necessarily want to hear about it*). We put ourselves into the shape of the sex we think we're supposed to be having, which is modeled on the example of a man's experience. We spend a lot of time in our heads, wondering if we're doing it right, concentrating very hard on "getting somewhere"—"somewhere" being synonymous with "climax." We think about what sounds we should be making while we're getting there, whether they're "right" or not. We wonder what our partner will think if we're not communicating via the aforementioned sounds that we're having a mind-blowingly rocking time. And what if the elusive climax never happens? In moments of desperation, or sheer exhaustion, we're sometimes tempted to fake it. Why not? Some of us feel like we're faking the whole thing anyway, starting with our interest in having sex in the first place. The result is that we distance ourselves from our desires, from our direct experience of sex, and in the end, from our orgasm. Some women have gotten so far away from their own authentic orgasm that they don't even think they *have* one. Which is a major concern, since <u>for women</u> <u>especially, *frequent access to the pleasure of orgasm is the*</u> <u>*key to finding joy, nourishment, and sustainable happiness*</u>. (How's that for a statement you don't hear every day?)

> "I've always been a sexual person, but for a long time I didn't feel like it was appropriate for me as a woman to have a really intense sexual appetite. So I ended up focusing on the guy's experience instead of my own. I got really good at performing. I would think, 'Oh, we're fucking. Does he like it? Should I do this or that?' But Slow Sex has changed that. It's helped me feel each sensation, to notice where I get scared, or when I start to pull away."
>
> —Margaret

So what's the solution to the problem of sex? While I was lucky enough to have Grandma teaching me in the kitchen, we don't have many artistic role models to look to in the bedroom. We are taught sex-as-science from the time we first stumble, fatally embarrassed, through sex ed. It continues right up through adulthood, where we can buy a sex manual for every problem (cementing the notion of sex-as-TV-repair) and fancy accoutrements to dress our little problem child up in. But there are very few <u>sexual</u> <u>mentors</u> floating around, slowly <u>reteaching the Art of Sex</u> to world-weary scientists.

"Very few indeed," I tell my now-wide-eyed students on that first day of class. "But lucky for you, you just found one."

A Note on the Exercises in This Book

The exercises throughout this book will ask you to let your sex come out and play—in full view of your partner, with the lights on. My students often look at me like I'm crazy when I tell them to turn toward their partners and simply begin talking about their sexual desire, right here, in the room with a whole bunch of other couples. Am I *mad*?

Maybe, maybe not. What I *am* doing is trying to unfreeze this idea we have that sex is a Very Serious Matter. To drop the recipe we usually use, one that calls for speed, diligence, and the lights being decidedly *off*. At its heart, you might say that's what Slow Sex is all about: turning the lights back on so we can all see what we're doing. There's no doubt it requires some students to step a bit outside of their comfort zones at first. Not a problem. Over the years I've watched in wonder as nervous, embarrassed students give themselves permission to let their sexual selves come out and play. Within a matter of seconds, wallflowers come into full bloom as wild, sexy beings they themselves have never seen before. It can happen for you, too. Just have fun with it! In my workshops I invite each student to approach the exercises I give them, and even the practice of Orgasmic Meditation itself, with the spirit of experimentation and play. You're researching your own experience of sex. What do you like? What could you do without? What did you feel in your body? What were you thinking about? Something about approaching sex as research lightens up the experience and makes it less capital "S" serious. It opens you up to play, to checking out this experience or that one, just because you're curious.

At the start of each exercise I've included the supplies you will need, including whether you'll need your partner for the exercise, and about how long it will take to complete. There are three exceptions, however. In addition to Orgasmic Meditation itself and other exercises that allow you to practice different aspects of Slow Sex, I have also included three exercises designed to help you translate the philosophy of Slow Sex into your "regular" sex life. These exercises—Slow Oral for Her, Slow Oral for Him, and Slow Intercourse, all found in chapter 8—are less about step-by-step instruction than inspiration. The exercises are intended to ignite a feeling inside of you, a feeling of what Slow Sex is really about. Sink deeply into the sensation they generate when you read them, and use the feeling—rather than the form—to guide you.

Exercise. Sex as a Science, Sex as an Art

This first exercise is a great place to start playing. You and your partner are going to test-drive sex as a science, and then sex as an art. It's meant to be fun and even a little bit saucy. How far you go is entirely up to you; you can change your mind or ask for something different at any moment. So give yourself permission to explore the unexplored and express whatever comes up with as little censorship as possible.

You'll need three pillows, your partner, and a journal(s) for this exercise.

Place the pillows in a triangle on top of the bed or on the floor. Choose one pillow to be the "science" seat, one to be the "art" seat, and one pillow just for "listening." Park your partner on the listening pillow. His job is simply to listen as you let your sex speak, and not get too hot and bothered to stay seated. Don't feel self-conscious making him do all the listening—he'll have his turn to talk soon enough!

Start by getting comfy on the science pillow, taking a minute to settle into your body and gather your attention. Then set your intention to research sex as science. Think linear, rational, goal-oriented, detailed, and even mathematical.

Now open your mouth and, using the most scientifically precise language you can muster, give your partner a quantitative recipe for fulfilling your sexual desire. Lay out exact instructions for how you want him to fuck you, with as much specificity as possible. What exactly do you want? Where? How often? For how long?

An example might be, "I want you to find me in the kitchen as I'm preparing dinner on Tuesday night. I want you to push me against the counter, lift up my skirt, and go down on me, alternating between sucking and licking my clit, while tugging firmly on my right nipple."

Maybe you have a fantasy you've always wanted him to fulfill—great, narrate it for him. Maybe you have never really thought about anything like this before—no problem, just start talking and see what comes out. Don't worry if you start laughing (humor is good!) or get embarrassed (remember, he's going next!). Keep talking as long as you have something to say.

As your flow of ideas winds down, move over to the "art" pillow. Once again, take a deep breath and gather your attention. You're in the world of art now—nonlinear, intuitive, emotional, and sensational.

When you're ready, start describing the *qualitative* feel of the sex you desire. Use motion, emotion, and even sound. Give him all the sensual details. You might say, "I want to feel you all the way inside of me, opening me up from the darkest, deepest corners. I want to feel the heaviness of your body

30

pinning me down, slow and unwavering, fucking the places I've never been touched before."

Whew—I'm getting hot just thinking about it!

Once the flow of ideas slows down, move back to the science perspective and continue speaking your desire, once again using quantitative language. Make sure all the details are on the table. When you feel complete, make one last stop on the art pillow and continue to paint him a portrait of what your desire looks, feels, tastes, and sounds like. Don't stop until you've said everything your desire wants to say.

Let your partner know when you are finished; then, take another moment to breathe and let everything you just said settle in the room. Ask your partner to mirror back to you what he heard you saying. He will then write down your desires from both the scientific perspective and the artistic perspective. (Feel free to help jog his memory if required.)

Once he is finished taking notes, switch positions. Take the listening seat, and have your partner complete the same exercise, starting with sex as science and moving on to sex as art.

When he is finished, be sure to record what you heard him say for future use.

Then have sex. You know you want to.

Advanced Practice

Plan four dates with your partner where you reenact the desires that arose during the exercise. (You have the notes: don't forget to study!) The dates may be as short as fifteen minutes or as long as a day or night. At the first date, your partner will enact your scientific desires; at the second, you will enact his. Take note of how much sensation, turn-on, and attention you have when you are engaging in "sex as science." Did everything turn out the way you expected? Did you feel as satisfied as you hoped when it was over? Take time to write in your journal about what you felt and how your expectations were or were not met.

Dedicate the next two dates to your artistic desires; first yours, then his. Invite the sensory details you described to come alive between you. Again, write down your experience in your journal. What did you feel? What turned you on? What had you feeling connected to your partner? Make time to share your thoughts and feelings with your partner. Remember to have fun—it's just sex, after all!

Sex Problems? No Such Thing

So now my students are becoming more relaxed and comfortable. They're on board that the way they've been handling the problem of sex is not working. Sex should be an art, not a science. Check. So now they're ready for me to start talking about how the "sex artist" solves the problem of sex.

Which is the first problem. It can't be done, I tell them. Simply put, *there is no solving the problem of sex.*

And with that, the relaxation gets sucked right back out of the room again. If there's no solving the problem of sex, then why on earth are they here? They want *solutions.* They were promised a *technique.* They want to know how any woman can be orgasmic in fifteen minutes—did I not read my own marketing materials? Throats begin to tighten; I think I see the guy in the corner turning blue. Life-saving measures are needed, stat.

"Problems are for scientists!" I blurt out. "Sex is an art,

remember? Therefore...?" I look around expectantly, waiting for someone to make the connection.

I'm getting crickets.

"*Therefore*," I fill in, "sex is not a problem."

We've been living with the paradigm of "wrong" for so long—with the mind-set that what is not flowing quote-unquote "smoothly," what is not unfolding as it "should" be, is wrong, a problem. But if I may say so, the paradigm of wrong is itself wrong! All you need to do in order to see that things don't always go the way you expect is to look at the world around you. Life is an all-inclusive package. You might think you paid only for joy/success/perfection, but like it or not, sadness/failure/inconsistency comes with the purchase price. "Wrong" is sometimes just part of the deal. Until we accept that fact—which holds up in the bedroom as well as everywhere else in life, BTW—we'll be running around like chickens with our heads cut off, chasing the good experiences and trying to avoid the bad ones. (A futile effort if I've ever seen one.) The irony is that the more we try to hang on to our best-ever sexual experiences for dear life, the more the not-so-good ones stick out. And the more we resist our sex problems, the more irritating/frustrating/painful they become. They start to take up a lot of energy—energy we might otherwise be putting toward other things.

Like, say, more orgasmic, more connected, more pleasurable sex. Yes?

No wonder we start to think that there's such a thing as "sex problems."

So the question is not how can we solve the *problems* that come along with sex, but instead, how can we extend and increase the pleasurable experiences we love, while coming to terms with all the other stuff, too? How do we at least make a truce with things like disappointment and failure and a sense of disconnection, so we can spend our time enjoying orgasmic bliss and deep connection and everything else that sex has to offer us?

The answer is Slow Sex, and the practice of Orgasmic Meditation. OM *does* offer a solution, and technically it *is* a technique. But what it's not is a recipe. It makes no promises about solving so-called sex problems, because in OM, there are no such things as problems, no such thing as hiding from the difficulties or clinging to the good times like a life preserver. By stripping away any expectations we have about what sex should or shouldn't be, teaching us how to pay attention to our own sensation, and encouraging honest and frequent communication with our partner, OM teaches us how to enjoy *all* the facets of our sexuality.

Unlike a science, when you decide to OM you're not getting any guarantees about the outcome. The only thing guaranteed is that, if you follow the instructions and really approach it with an open mind, you will end up an artist. You will become reacquainted with your own personal muse: your own genuine orgasm. Your tools will be your partner, your own body, and your desire. Your only job is to pay attention. There, in that moment of listening, of using your desire as a compass, you go from experiencing sex as a science to sex as an art. That is the switch that turns the lights on. It's what your sex life is asking for.

The result—the reward you will get for this radical act of relaxation—is freedom. Freedom from all the pressure that usually accompanies sex. Men, especially, are freed from the constant pressure that sex, and particularly their partner's orgasm, needs to be "figured out." The sheer simplicity of the OM practice, and the fact that no particular outcome is expected, relegates their fixing mind to the back burner. Women, for our part, are freed from the narrow definition of "orgasmic" that we've been confined to ever since we learned what sex was about. Instead of forging ahead toward a climax as it is traditionally defined, our every experience, our every sensation, becomes part of our orgasm. This last point cannot be overstated. For re-envisioning our definition of "orgasm"—modeling it on the nuance of female orgasm, rather than the goal orientation of male orgasm—allows all of us, men and women alike, to draw more complete nourishment from our sex.

~

After starting to practice OM, you can't help but have a completely different definition of orgasm. Whereas once we thought of orgasm as an "intensely pleasurable moment in time, which, if done right, provides satisfaction and release," suddenly it can also be an "intensely pleasurable period of time, which, regardless of outcome, offers the opportunity for revolutionary connection and transformational enjoyment." (Catchy, no?) The former definition is the more straightforward male model of orgasm—which we still love. But when we OM, we also get to know the more female model. It may not look as glamorous at first, but it gives us a whole lot of something else—something we've been looking for.

A Note to My Same-Sex Friends

My Slow Sex workshops are full of students from all walks of life, including—and perhaps especially—all sexual orientations. Regardless of whether you sleep with men, women, or some combination of both, the principles of Slow Sex are the same. For reasons that I will discuss later, however, beginning OM practice focuses primarily on a man stroking a woman. For this reason, the language in this book will be primarily hetero-focused. That said, for my gay male readers, there *is* a male stroking practice, which you'll start hearing about in chapter 3. For my lesbian friends, the traditional OM practice is still perfectly applicable, though contrary to my instruction for hetero couples, you may consider trading off stroking duties. That way you both receive the benefits of being stroked, which, as women, is the key to uncovering our own unique orgasm.

The transition from traditional sex toward Slow Sex is similar to other transformations that are happening all around us. Take exercise, for example. You might say that OM is to "conventional sex" what yoga is to more conventional exercise, like aerobics. With aerobics—or running, or most other forms of exercise—there is often (but not always) some sort of quantitative goal involved. You might work out to build strength and stamina, lose weight, or just clear your head. The stated goal of yoga, however, is simply to stay with your breath. The practice itself is to let go of any expectations about outcome. Falling out of the posture is just as much a part of the experience as nailing an arm balance for the first time. That's what makes yoga an art form. It's different every time you try it. And every time you learn something new, get a new appreciation for who you are and what you're capable of.

This is not to say that you can't still enjoy a good, hard

workout on its own merit. Exercise for the benefit of exercise will always have its place. But through yoga, a different possibility has entered the mix—the possibility of strengthening body and mind while also contacting something deeper inside of ourselves.

In the same way, OM is not intended to be a replacement for sex. On the contrary, most people practice Slow Sex because of how much it improves their "regular" sex lives. But like yoga, OM shows us a whole different world is available. A world where there are no such things as "sex problems." Where what matters is not the outcome, but the pleasure you receive along the way. The best news? The skills we develop through Slow Sex act like rocket fuel when we apply them to traditional sex.

The benefits of OM only make themselves known, however, when we approach the practice like art instead of science. Anyone who has unrolled her yoga mat with the idea that she's going to nail a particular posture knows that approaching your yoga practice with a goal in mind is just asking for a piece of humble pie. Demand of yourself that you're going to nail side plank and watch yourself fall out of position before you even get there. In fact, in yoga they say that success is just getting to the mat in the first place. OM is the same way. Deciding you want to practice *is* the practice. Feeling the first stroke is the practice. Everything else is like icing on the cake. Like any art form, the path will be different every time. Sometimes it's boring, frustrating, irritating. Other times it's mind-blowing, heart-opening, and hot. The former is just as much a victory as the latter. What you will learn is how to stay open for both.

This is not to say you can't spend time investigating the possibility of sex as a science. Hey, if that's what you want to do, I say go for it. There are plenty of sex manuals out there that will teach you positioning, technique, etiquette, and how to have and give a conventional climax every time. But these books are like the recipes I learned in Home Ec class. They explain sex from the outside in, rather than teaching you how to experience sex from the inside out. This book, and the practice of OM, is about the art. You'll get a core technique, but in this world, technique will only take you so far. I'll let you in on a bunch of sex secrets I've learned over the years, but after that the ball is in your court. It's what *you* put into it that counts.

The good news is that Slow Sex simplifies things. It throws out all expectation about what her orgasm should look like and how he is going to give it to her. It takes the pressure off, for both men and women. It makes room for everyone and every possibility. Whether you've ever had a traditional climax or not, orgasm awaits you.

One more confession, which you've probably already surmised. This book is about sex, sure. But on a different level, this book is actually about *your life*. It's about learning a new way of operating in the world, which in turn allows for new ways of relating to other people and your life as a whole. It's about putting down roots. Learning how to feel your own body. Learning how to connect with other people. And it's about letting go of expectations and instead making room for every possibility. In a nutshell, this book is about turning your life into a work of art. It just so happens that the medium we're going to be using— the magic potion that will get you there—is sex. Because if there's one thing I've discovered on my own journey, it's that sex is like New York: if you can make it there, you can make it *anywhere*.

"With the OMing practice I'm able to really feel what's inside of me. I love what's inside of me, and I want to feel more and more and more. My orgasm really comes out during OM. Then, when I'm having sex, I'm feeling more all the time. Which is a relief, because my biggest fear was that I wouldn't ever be able to feel sex again."

—Annika, 37

Now, don't get me wrong. If straight-up *better sex* is what you're looking for, Slow Sex offers that, too. It's one of the side effects of coming back into your body and into relationship with your world. When you strip sex down, pay attention to sensation, and ask for what you desire, you can expect richer, more satisfying orgasms; a deeper, more nourishing connection with your partner; and improved relationships with everyone in your life. In just a few minutes a day, you can learn how to live—how to make the most of your one and precious life! How you can get inside it, be a part of it, feel intimate with the world in a whole new way. It's a promise I've seen come to fruition in the lives of too many students to count. I know the same is available here for you, too, no matter who you are or why you're here.

Chapter Two

The Three Ingredients for Slow Sex

Now, about that technique...?"

Enough with the philosophy! If you're like most of my students, you're ready to hear the details of the practice by now. Which is only natural, after all. When we hear the term "sex practice," we automatically assume we're talking about an unusual position or outlandish technique. Not for nothing; we live in a "more is better" culture. When things need a lift in the bedroom, we've been taught that the answer is to add something to the experience—toys, sexy talk, lingerie, tantric postures, massage oils, you name it. When I put our little OM technique out there as something truly new and different, our minds head toward fireworks and cannonballs. What on earth could OM be all about? How crazy/strange/titillating/FUN is this practice going to be, given that she's billing it as *better* than sex toys?

Alas, the first "ingredient" in OM practice—<u>stripping down all our expectations</u>—comes into play right at the beginning, before most students have even started the practice. Because by comparison to what we *think* we're going to be getting with a "sex practice," the step-by-step instruction for OM can appear underwhelming. There will be no fireworks here, just one very light, very subtle stroke. And there is much less physical contact—and significantly less nudity—than students expect. In fact, I can summarize the entire practice in just one paragraph:

OM is most often practiced between a man and a woman. The woman removes her clothes from the waist down. She lies down on a bed or the floor and butterflies her legs open. Her partner places a pillow under each of her knees for support. He sits to her left, with his left leg over her belly and his right leg under her knees, where he can both see and access her genitals. Once in position, he looks at her genitals and describes in a few words what he sees. He then applies lube to his left forefinger and starts to stroke the sensitive left side of her clitoris using a very light touch. He continues to stroke for fifteen minutes, during which time both partners place their attention on the point of connection between them. The stroker may ask the receiver yes-or-no questions and adjust the pressure and direction of his stroke based on her feedback and the sensation he himself is feeling in his body. When the fifteen minutes is up, he grounds the sexual energy that has built up in her body by pressing the palm of one hand firmly against her clit for a few seconds. Then each partner shares a "frame," or a description of one particularly memorable moment of sensation they felt while OMing. The practice can be done as often as you like, but I suggest a regular practice of three to five times per week.

"It sounds like OMing is more like meditation than it is like sex," I often hear after revealing the details. To my students' chagrin, I nod enthusiastically. Yes. That's exactly it.

Some disappointment is natural. We've gotten so conditioned to be looking for *more* rather than less. We would never think that simplification is the key, that we'll find more satisfaction when we *subtract* rather than add. So much for the sexiness of Slow Sex; subtraction never got anyone a first date. We are an acquisition culture, always wanting more and better and new and different. Cars, houses, wives—you name it, we add it. Subtraction is invited only when it makes room for us to add something else.

But as I mentioned earlier, Slow Sex is like Slow Food. The first step in Slow Sex is to strip down to the essentials. In Slow Food, this means starting with fresh, organic, local produce and sustainably raised meats. True flavor becomes the main event. In Slow Sex, the main event is sensation. There's no involved interpretation, no accoutrements, just bare sensation. We strip away everything until all we have left is two people, their nerve endings, and a light but precise stroke. That's where it all begins.

The most radical part of starting OM with sensation is that we have to let go of all the other baggage we've been carrying around. Since it doesn't look anything like our normal idea of sex—it's not intercourse, it's not oral sex, and the guy doesn't even take off his clothes—we are no longer confined to our expectations of what sex and orgasm should look like. And since the stroke is performed almost exclusively on the woman, we get to see a whole different version of orgasm than the one we're used to.

A version that's about the journey rather than the destination. A version that's softer and more nuanced—slower

42

and more relaxing. A version that may or may not include a conventional climax.

A version that can last an hour. Or four hours. Or four *months.*

Slow Sex doesn't look so boring anymore, does it?

It's true: by the time you finish this book you'll know everything you need to know to have a four-month orgasm. There are no tools required—just three simple ingredients. *1)* First, you'll have to take it all off: be willing to strip sex down to the barest essentials, adding nothing extra. Second, *2)* you'll have to learn how to pay attention to the sensations in your body, feeling them, naming them, and returning to them over and over. Finally, you have to be willing to com- *3)* municate freely and openly with your partner—including and especially asking for what you really want every step of the way. (Which requires you to *know* what you really want—which, never fear, is a by-product of ingredients one and two.)

Three basic ingredients. Sounds simple enough in theory, I realize, but in practice it's not always so.

That's okay—that's why I'm here. To walk you through, every step of the way. In OM we call this "safeporting." Safeporting is the practice of telling your partner everything you are about to do before you actually do it. Safeporting means everyone can relax and feel the stroke without fear of what's coming next. This is especially important for women. Studies have shown that during orgasm, a man's brain lights up mainly in the pleasure centers. But when a woman enters an orgasmic state, several major areas of her brain go silent—particularly those involved with inhibition, appropriateness, and evaluating her environment for possible threats. Because of this phenomenon, a sense of safety is an absolute prerequisite for a woman to lower her guard enough to really get off. So, safeport her. After all, the only surprises we want during OM are the orgasmic kind, and believe me, if I know anything about orgasm, there are a whole lot of surprises in store. (For instructions on safeporting during the OM, see chapter 3.)

Stripping Down

A couple of years ago, we needed to redesign the interior of our OneTaste retreat center in San Francisco. Over the course of time we had accumulated so much furniture, in so many different styles and colors, that the place was starting to look like a garage sale. Our classes were getting big enough that we were at the breaking point: the clutter had to go or we'd have to start seating people on the bookshelves.

I called in my friend Marta. Now, I knew from spending time in Marta's home and office that she understood design. She is, in fact, an incredibly good interior designer. But when she started by telling everyone to carry all the furniture from inside the center out onto the sidewalk, I got panicky. First, we're in the heart of San Francisco here, and in a big city like that furniture sitting on the street is fair game. Second, shouldn't a designer have vision? Shouldn't she be able to rearrange things in a space without having to clear it out completely?

So I parked myself on one of the couches outside, ready to slap the hand of anybody who even looked sideways at my furniture, and watched as Marta instructed the OneTaste staff to bring the furniture back inside, one piece at a time.

About an hour later, after they'd moved just two-thirds of the center's contents back inside, Marta came out and announced they were done. Done? What about the couch I was sitting on? Where was that going to go?

Marta gently guided me away from the couch and ushered me into the center. Which had, in the span of one hour, become an entirely different space. It was like someone had come in and bathed the whole center in sparkly sunlight. Everything was the same, but the relationship between the furniture and the room—and the way the place *felt*—was completely different. It was as if every chair, table, and couch had grown organically, up from the very floor and presented itself in its perfect location. The negative space in between (and there was such spaciousness, so much warm and inviting space!) was as welcoming as the cozy nooks and intimate relationships she'd created between the pieces of furniture. It was as if this whole different world had been there all along, just waiting for us to uncover it.

OM is to sex what Marta was to the center: it clears out all the sexual furniture we've accumulated and then brings back only the pieces that are the most sensational. When we OM, we strip sex down far enough that it doesn't even look like "sex" anymore—and then we feel our way back in. We let go of everything we've ever been taught about orgasm, male/female roles, and how sex is "supposed" to look, and replace it with what *feels* good and right and pleasurable.

OM is our get-out-of-jail-free card, cleaning the slate and letting us start over from scratch. What would sex look like if we had never been taught how to do it? What does orgasm look like if we let go of our previous definitions? If it doesn't *have* to be this ultimate, mind-blowing experience of "going over," then what *might* it be? What deeper pleasure might we be able to find within it? With that much freedom, what infinite possibilities exist beyond our wildest imagination?

Taking It All Off

Slow Sex is about simplicity. It is about discovering just how much orgasmic sensation is available during sex—sensation we usually miss out on because we're spending so much energy adding to the experience. If there's one thing you take away from this book, I hope it's the knowledge that orgasm doesn't need your help! You don't have to trust me on that—all you have to do is OM. When you strip away everything extra, the power of your own authentic orgasm will say it all. To that end, here are just a few things I recommend leaving behind while you start practicing Slow Sex:

Expectations. In Slow Sex, we make a conscious decision to experience our sex just as it is, every single time, without anything added—not even our expectations. No expectation for climax, for fireworks, even for a "good" experience versus a "bad" one. Nothing but a natural sense of curiosity.

The Harder-and-Faster Mentality. Porn-style thrashing is to sex what air guitar is to rock music—a whole lot of show and not much substance. The best sex is the kind where you don't want to move an inch. In Slow Sex, we nix the habit of trying to increase sensation by increasing speed and pressure. Instead, when we feel sensation decrease, we apply more attention. Rather than trying to add something, we look more and more carefully at what is already there.

→ Vibrators. I always feel bad about mentioning this, because I know how fun and effective vibrators can be. But the unfortunate truth is that they are also hard on a woman's tender parts. They give a lot of pressure to a very wide area, and the result is that they tend to numb sensation in the clit itself. If you are willing to set them aside, at least for a period, you will discover that the steady, subtle OM stroke can draw your clit back to life. As its eight thousand nerve endings begin to fire again, you won't believe the amount of sensation you will be able to access. You may never need to pick up your vibrator again.

→ Fantasy. Many women I meet create elaborate fantasy worlds where they retreat during sex. Many men, for their part, spend a lot of time with porn. Role playing, sexy lingerie— there are hundreds of ways we bring fantasy into our sex. We've gotten so used to it that many of us don't think we can get off without these additions. The problem is that fantasy is a way we step *out* of our experience of sex, rather than stepping further *into* it. When I say that Slow Sex is about letting go of everything extra, I am including the safety blanket of fantasy. Putting all our attention on sensation instead allows us to go as deeply as possible into the sex we're actually having, right now.

→ Romance. I hate to even bring this up because it makes me feel like the Grinch Who Stole Christmas. So let me say up front that there is *nothing wrong* with romance. I love romance. The problem is, however, that we've bought into the idea that romance is required for us to access the deepest levels of sexual nourishment. Sex must be with someone we love; the relationship has to be "going some-where"; our partner has to prove their love for us by gazing, Hollywood-style, into our eyes. Unfortunately, when you set these storyline requirements for sex, you end up back at the top of this list: with a whole lot of expectations. Slow Sex calls us to connect with another person at a level even more essential than a romantic storyline—at the level of what is, right now. It may be romantic, and it may not. But at least it's real.

Your Attention, Please

If stripping down is the first ingredient in Slow Sex, then the second is paying attention. Paying attention is essential to great art, great lovemaking, and great OM. Unfortunately, attention tends to be in short supply when it comes to sex. When it comes to life, for that matter. The reason is twofold: First, our on-the-go world doesn't place much value on noticing, listening, and feeling. Paying attention isn't going to get us anywhere, and going somewhere is what we've been told we're supposed to be doing. All the time. Bored? Go *do* something! Feeling stuck, depressed, or just generally out of sorts? Go exercise, go have sex, go eat something, go shopping. These messages have entered our psyche deeply enough that many of us actually feel guilty when we're *not* doing something. We are a society that doesn't let grass grow beneath our feet—even if watching the grass grow is exactly what we want to do on any given afternoon. There is very little support in our world for just taking the time to *be*. We have been conditioned against being the kind of person who just *is*.

The second reason we don't pay attention to our sex is that we aren't that good at it. Life in our time is a noisy place to be. We've got advertising screaming at us all day long; we've got TV and hard rock and the roar of traffic. With all this ruckus, how are we supposed to hear the subtle cues, the fine-tuned messages, that want to come through—especially during sex? Many of my students don't even believe there *is* such a thing. I talk about listening to the space, listening to our sex, and my students are ready to pack up their things and go. They didn't sign up for any New Age claptrap and here I go, asking them to listen to things that—let's see, how can I put this gently?— *don't talk*.

I don't get offended. In our loud and frantic world, such attention is in limited supply. And yet attention is required if you're going to become an artist, of sex or anything else. It is the fairy dust that turns straw into gold, the way you turn up the volume so you can hear your world talking to you. But unless you were raised by Buddhist monks and left in a cave to contemplate the tip of your nose for the first couple decades of your life, you probably don't have much practice cultivating attention. I demonstrate this fact in class by conducting a simple exercise. I give each student a beautiful flower and tell them to pay attention to it for ninety seconds. No need to think anything particular about it—they're not going to be asked to describe it later, there will be no quiz. They're only to observe the flower.

When the exercise is over, I ask the students whether the flower was more vibrant at the beginning of the exercise or at the end. Every single hand goes up for "at the beginning." I don't think I've ever had a student answer differently. Over time—even just over the course of a minute and a half—our attention wanes. This seems normal, doesn't it? It happens all the time. The day you hang a new painting on the wall, it's all you see when you walk into the room. By day three, you barely notice it anymore. Same thing happens in relationship: at the beginning of a relationship you are euphoric, and your new love is literally all you can think about. Check back three years later, and the situation is likely to have settled. You're used to having her around, and as much as you may still love her, your attention has moved on to other things. It's inevitable.

Or is it? I am going to make a big statement in saying that it is *not* inevitable. Attention is a skill we can develop as much or as little as we choose. Should you choose to develop yours—say, through the practice of OM, just as an example—you will see that there is no limit to its possibility. Attention makes everything around us better. Relationships can become more and more enjoyable day by day. Sexual interest can grow, rather than wane, over time. And OM is the best way I know to develop sustainable attention. I'm going to take a big position here: you can't have great sex without sustainable attention. Not just because you won't be there to know whether you're having great sex or not, which you won't. But actually because attention is the special sauce. Attention makes sex exponentially better. It's like salting your food. Ever wonder why a bland meal magically comes to life with just a pinch of salt? Me, too. How does salt *do* it? Attention does the same thing. Think of it as salt for sex. For reasons that do not make themselves immediately clear, a pinch of attention can turn previously tasteless sex into a gourmet meal. It can get you into relationship with your partner and yourself and what you're doing right now.

"When you said I needed to be listening to my sex, I thought I was in big trouble," more than one student has explained. "I have been told I can't even listen to my wife."

Not to worry. OM itself is an excellent way to learn the art of listening. The upside is that you're going to be able to unlock the secrets of the universe. The downside is that once you have more attention to spare, there will be no more excuses for not taking out the garbage.

The Power of Sensation

So you're game to give this old attention-cultivation thing a try. But what is it, exactly, that you're going to be paying attention to? You want to learn how to listen, but what are you supposed to be listening to? The answer is *sensation*. Sensation is the star of the show, both in sex and in life. In fact, I would argue that it's our primary motivation for just about everything. We want money so we can buy the sensations of luxury, security, status, and even the ability to help others. We want relationship because we desire the sensations of sex, and companionship, as well as being seen and understood. We usually think of these desires as external circumstances or internal emotions, but in fact, all of them correspond to feelings in the body—sensations.

"Why do I OM? The one word that comes up is '*desire*.' I have always had a desire to get more out of sex. And that's what I got when I started OMing, when I learned how to connect to my sensation at the most basic level. I just feel *more* when I OM."   —Tom, 56

Sensations are perceived using one or more of our five senses. The smell of a beautiful flower is a sensation, as is the taste of a decadent piece of chocolate. With a few exceptions, when we're talking about sensation in the context of sex we're talking about our sense of touch. Touch goes deeper than feeling something with our fingers—anything you feel in your body is coming through your sense of touch. You know you're hungry because you feel the sensation of hunger in your belly; you know you just stepped on a thorn because you feel the sensation of pain in your foot. And of course, you know you are attracted to someone when you feel the sensations of arousal. The sensations of arousal are different for everyone, but they might include a feeling of heat centralized in the genitals, a feeling of pleasure expanding throughout your body, and more. These are all experienced through your sense of touch.

What you may not understand yet is how tricky this territory actually is. Sensation sounds easy enough, but you'd be surprised how difficult it is for most of my new students to name even one sensation they are feeling in their bodies right this very moment. There's a tendency to cross-reference sensation with our "feelings"—to name an emotion rather than a sensation. What I'm looking for is something like "A heavy, flattened feeling under my thighs as I sit in this chair." What I often hear instead is something like "happiness" or "anxiety" or "annoyance." The former is sensation—something felt with the sense of touch. The latter is emotion—an interpretation of what sensation *means*.

It's not as if most of us have much experience naming our sensations. Even if we can identify one—say, that dense, dark, fluttery sensation that's kind of below the heart but toward the back, maybe near the left kidney—we don't necessarily have the words to express it. After all, we grow up trying to push away a lot of our sensations, particularly those we've categorized as "negative." From the first day of school when we announce the feeling of butterflies in our stomachs and are immediately told that we're "just feeling nervous," we are taught to reframe sensation as emotion. While the two are obviously related—nerves often do result in a fluttery feeling in the stomach—the message we're getting is that when we feel sensation, the next step is interpretation. The sensation itself is not really worth discussing. Instead, when we feel something in the body, we either ignore it or retreat to the mind to reason ourselves back to comfort.

Like any other skill, if we don't use our feeling sense, we lose it. What we ignore tends to fade away. So most of us arrive in the world of Slow Sex and discover that our sensory detection system is out of order. And we wonder why we're not getting the sensation we desire from our sex lives! We're so out of practice that oftentimes neither the stroker nor the receiver feels very much when he or she is first starting to OM. The stroke is so fine—like the lightest of feathers—that it seems like "nothing is happening." I get a lot of cranky practitioners coming back after trying OM for the first time, saying that they just can't do it. This practice is not going to work for them—they're not getting anywhere.

My response is—fantastic! You've just made one of the biggest discoveries of your life, one that most people will never take the time to learn. You're recognizing that your sensory system has been underused, neglected, and even repressed. The very system that is motivating your life is completely out of order. It's why men have a hard time feeling their way when they're pleasuring a woman, why they can't access their own gut instinct about how to make her feel good every single time. And of course, it's why women have a hard time really sinking down into the experience of sex—without access to their own sensations, how are they supposed to feel sex and know their own orgasm? Not to mention to extract the enjoyment and nourishment they crave from it, that they know is available but can't seem to access.

But don't lose heart—now that you know what's gone awry, there's hope! It's like people who say they can't do yoga because they aren't flexible enough, or people who say they can't meditate because their mind keeps wandering. The whole point of yoga is to develop flexibility. The whole point of meditation is to develop your attention skills. And the whole point of OM—or one of them, anyway—is to cultivate the ability to feel. To feel your sexuality, your sensations, and your world, starting with what's happening in your body right now.

"I had gotten to the point where I didn't think I was a sexual person anymore. I hadn't felt any sort of sex drive for years. At first I couldn't feel his stroke at all when we OMed, but over the course of the first few weeks I started to feel a little more and then a little more. And then that same feeling started to translate to regular sex. I found myself actually looking forward to sex for the first time in as long as I can remember."   —Shari, 51

It's easy to see why we're so addicted to addition. What we want in life is more and more sensation, right? But since so few of us have working sensation detection systems, the natural tendency is to want to add more and more until we *can* feel something. It's like someone who is losing their hearing and starts turning up the volume on the TV. Pretty soon you've got the thing on so loud that the window-panes are vibrating and the dog is hiding under the bed. Rather than increasing attention, most of us opt to increase the noise. We don't have enough attention to keep sensation vibrant (remember the flower exercise?) so we keep adding more and more and more sensation in hopes of recapturing the experience of seeing the flower for the first time. We've grown used to roses so we breed ever bigger varieties, with ever more enormous blooms, in ever more fantastic colors. We've grown used to our partners so we add new sex positions and eye-gazing practices and toys and porn to help get ourselves in the mood again. The problem is that this strategy never works. No matter how outlandish our sex becomes, without cultivating our attention and our ability to feel sensation, we'll eventually be numb to even the most radical sexual practices. Instead, we need to get back to basics. Get our attention burning brighter and then use it to experience the pure sensations available in our bodies all the time. It's the only way to make sex sustainable—not to mention that it's a whole lot less traumatic for the dog.

Exercise. Listening to Your Body During Sex

Sex is one of the most fun, most exciting, and most satisfying activities available on planet Earth—so why do so many of us check out completely while it's going on? We're in our heads, or thinking about what we'll cook for dinner, or caught up in a fantasy that has little to nothing to do with what's going on in our bodies in the present moment. Whatever our particular brand of zoning out, for most of us the experience is the same. We're not observing—and thus not enjoying—the fireworks display of pure physical sensation that is happening in our very own bodies.

So here's your assignment: the next time you are engaged in a sexual encounter (whether with another person or flying solo), set the intention to simply *feel the sensation in your genitals*. This may sound remedial—isn't that what we do when we have sex, we feel our genitals? But if you're like most of us, you'll discover the surprising truth that you have been spending most of your sex life thinking about everything *but* the feeling in your genitals. You've been thinking about your partner's experience, or how long an orgasm is taking, or about the celebrity you always think about when you're having sex. Instead, this one time, pay attention to the sensation in your genitals.

Try to name at least one sensation you can feel. If you're practicing as a couple, describe the sensation to your partner. Use color, texture, motion, and location. Otherwise simply name the sensation you are feeling to yourself. Try to stay aware of your genitals for the rest of the encounter.

Practicing Orgasmic Meditation may not be the *only* way to retrain ourselves to feel sensation, but it's surely the most fun. It's also the most effective: there really isn't any more intense, more potent, more electric source of physical sensation we can access than our own sexuality. So why not start there? OM gets right to the heart of the matter, putting our most sensitive body parts to their very best use. There are a lot of other meditation practices out there, from basic breathing meditation to more embodied visualization practices, all of which can work very well for cultivating your attention. (For some recommendations, see Further Resources at the back of the book.) I should know, because I've tried them all. Before I found OM, I was about to throw in the towel on sex altogether and join a Zen monastery. But there was a little voice that kept nagging at the back of my mind. It said that for me, leaving my sexuality behind was never going to bring me the sensations I craved. The sensations of deep satisfaction, enjoyment, and aliveness. I knew the voice was right: for me, the skill of drawing enjoyment from every experience, in every moment of my life, could be learned only through sex. Maybe the same goes for you.

Asking for What You Desire

Looking back, it's kind of surprising that I listened to that voice, since at the time I could have rattled off a hundred different things I enjoyed doing more than I enjoyed having sex. Eating cookies, for one. Going to the movies, for another. Watching paint dry...

As much sex as I was having—and objectively, I was having quite a lot—I was very rarely getting joy out of it. I was hardly even *there* for it. I spent a whole lot of time pretending to be absorbed in orgasmic connection, while in reality I was doing all sorts of other things in my head. Making to-do lists. Thinking about what I was going to cook for dinner. Wondering how much longer he was going to take...

In other words, sex—the most sensational, exciting, spectacular experience we can have in the human body—was not sensational, exciting, or spectacular enough to hold my attention.

It took my finding Orgasmic Meditation to really understand what was going on. Sure, it had to do with the fact that I hadn't yet learned to *cultivate* my attention, much less to place it on the sensation in my body and then keep it there. (I've since discovered that if you can do that, even watching paint dry turns out to be a completely engrossing activity.) But it also had to do with something I was not willing to do. Something that happens to be the third key ingredient for Slow Sex but takes the prize as the number one hardest thing to actually *do* during sex, especially for women:

To ask for what we truly desire.

I don't know if it's some massive conspiracy or what, but somehow over the growing-up process women receive little positive reinforcement for speaking our desires. We're cautioned every step of the way to not voice our sexual desires, for fear of looking like a "bad woman," appearing too needy, stumbling down the supposedly slippery slope toward promiscuity, or—this is a big one—permanently damaging the supposedly fragile male ego. Whatever the reason, the result is that we women fall into patterns of pleasing others, especially during sex. By the time we're adults, and we actually *want* sexual satisfaction enough to ask for it, we find that a sort of desire paralysis has set in. We've kept our desires so well hidden that we don't even remember where we put them. I see this every time I teach a Slow Sex workshop and I ask women to talk about their desires.

"What desires?" one woman asks, and the rest nod in agreement. Lots of the women I meet don't think they even *have* desires anymore. It's like they tucked them away for safekeeping and now they can't remember where they put them. They locked them up in the "good girl" drawer, the mothering drawer, the sexual trauma drawer, the menopause drawer—and now they can't find the key.

At first. That's the good news. As most women discover over the course of their first few OMing sessions, their desires are closer than they think. All that time they were sure desire was dead and buried, it was actually hiding just beneath the surface, waiting for permission to take a few tentative steps out into the sunlight, to walk around and feel the grass under its feet. I can't wait to give desire that permission! I often go around the room in my workshop and ask each student to toss out just one thing that they want—just one little desire. The first student is hesitant, embarrassed, not sure if she's *really* allowed to reveal what she *really* wants. But as soon as she summons the courage to tell me something, one little thing, desires start poking their heads out all over the place. The class starts getting giddy, like a bunch of kids, shouting out their desires for more sex, more connection, more enjoyment, or for a triple-shot half-caff vanilla latte (it's usually a Saturday morning, after all). It's the sweetest thing to see my room full of mostly savvy, mostly urban, mostly "together" Slow Sex students regress back to younger, more carefree, more desirous versions of themselves. Sweet, but also poignant— since who they become during this exercise is usually the kid they were around about the time they learned to shove their desires in a drawer.

I first got that message myself when I was five or six. Whenever I saw a woman wearing a miniskirt—and it was the seventies, so I saw a lot of women wearing miniskirts— I would feel a driving desire to tiptoe up behind them, lean in, and sink my teeth deep into the backs of their knees. Needless to say, this did not go over so well with the ladies. My auntie Doris found it increasingly difficult to explain my odd little fetish to her friends at church, so one day when I went in for my signature move, she swatted me away. "Nicole," she said with seriousness. "You don't want to do that. You want to be a good girl."

I was pretty sure she was wrong; I was pretty sure I'd rather be biting women on the backs of their knees than being a good girl. But the shame I felt at being reprimanded burned hot on my cheeks and stayed with me for days. I never wanted to feel *that* again. So without further ado, I threw my knee-biting resources toward being a good girl.

In time, I was throwing nearly all of my resources there. So were you. So were we all. This is what happens when we're growing up: we're taught which desires are appropriate and which are not, and we become ashamed of anything in the latter category. In time all the shameful experiences grow into a big, heavy patchwork quilt. What we don't realize is that the quilt is still with us, lo these many years hence. We may think we threw it out a long time ago, but in truth all those memories of shame are still there, scaring the crap out of our desire. So the next exercise I give the students is designed to let their desire—their sexual desire in particular—enjoy some fresh air for a change.

Exercise. Taking Dictation from Your Sex

In the world of Slow Sex, there may be no lesson as mind-blowing as learning how to ask our partner for what we want. But first, we have to figure out what it *is* we want. That's where this exercise comes in. As I said previously, most of us have been keeping our desire, especially our sexual desire, on lock-down. In this exercise, you're going to reverse that trend. You're going to hand your desire the microphone—and then you're going to sit back and take dictation.

This is a writing exercise, so you'll need a quiet spot, a journal, a timer, and about fifteen minutes.

First, sit down and get comfortable. Feel your feet on the floor, your own weight as you sit quietly. Pay attention to which sensations you can feel in your body. If you notice any pain or tension, be aware of it for a few moments and then move on. Now identify three separate sensations, and speak or whisper them out loud. "My feet feel cool on the floor." "I can feel a sort of sparkly light sensation in the front of my chest." "My insides feel dark and wet and mossy green." Speaking your sensations is a great way to return to what's happening right now. Once you're finished, and you feel like you've really landed in your body, you're ready to begin.

Set your timer for eight minutes and get ready to write. You are going to answer the question "What does my sex want, right now?" When the timer starts, put your pen down on the page and don't pick it up again until the timer chimes. Start off with, "What my sex wants right now is..." And let your desire do the talking from there.

Try not to censor yourself—if your sex wants to get fucked, if it wants to be naughty, if it wants to do things your conscious mind would never have thought to do, let it have its say. You're not responsible for anything it says or does; your only job is to give it space to roam—and to take notes. If your desire takes you to a place that doesn't feel comfortable to you, never fear. You're not agreeing to actually *act on* this list—all you're agreeing to do is write it down.

If you become stuck at any point, just go back to "What my sex wants right now is..." Keep writing, even if you don't know what to write. Keep writing, even if you write, "What my sex wants right now is... *to know what my sex wants right now!*" That's actually a pretty interesting discovery in itself.

When the timer goes off, finish up the sentence you're on, then put down the pen. Re-read the essay on desire that you just wrote. Do you approve of what your sex wrote, or not? Did anything surprise you? Do you feel like you really let your sex have its say, or did you hold something back out of fear? What do the sensations in your body feel like after having let your desire run free for eight minutes? Did the exercise expand you, or do you feel more contracted? Are you feeling freer, or did you get embarrassed or anxious? There are no right answers here; it's all research, after all.

Advanced Practice

Ask your partner to do the above exercise along with you. When you are both finished writing, sit across from one another. Ask her to pay attention to the sensation in her body as you read your essay to her. Once you are finished reading, have her share one sensation she felt while you read. Once she has shared her sensation, invite her to read her essay to you while you pay attention to the sensation in your body. When she is finished reading, share one sensation you felt while listening to her desire speak.

Sometimes I think that if I had only one thing in the world I could teach, it would be the ability to identify our sexual desires and then learn how to ask for them. Especially for women, who have been shamed into hiding and repressing our hunger—sexual and otherwise—it can feel risky and dangerous to admit that we want something more or different from whatever it is we're currently getting. I once had a couple come to a coaching session and neither was happy with their collective sex life. He knew on some level he wasn't pleasing her, but she wouldn't tell him what to do differently. We discovered during the session that she didn't want to tell him what to do, because she was too afraid of hurting his feelings. So, she told me, she "just let it go."

"I kind of gave up on the idea of getting satisfied sexually, because he couldn't push my buttons and I just couldn't bring myself to tell him how," she said. "I can't believe I'm saying this, but I felt like it would be better to let our sex life die than to risk asking for what I wanted."

I hear this all the time, in many different ways. And although men definitely do experience some level of fear around asking for what they want, I find that this is much more of a problem for women. Both because—as previously discussed—women's bodies are more complicated, and also because women's *psyches* are more complicated. In this area, Orgasmic Meditation can have a huge impact. It makes asking for what we want a part of the practice itself. Nobody's feelings have to get hurt, because it's part of the script, so to speak.

> "Through OM, my relationship to sex has changed. I have more approval for what I desire, or things I want to try. Just because I want to try something doesn't mean I have to do it, it doesn't mean I'm a certain person—whatever judgment I have about people who do this kind of thing—it just means some part of me might want to have this experience once. Putting a desire out there doesn't make it a request. It doesn't even mean that you'll do anything about it. It's just feeling free enough to say 'I want this.'"
> —Hillary, 32

The best part is that once you build the muscle of asking for what you desire during sex, you can flex it in the rest of your life as well. A new student of mine was telling me how the most amazing moment of her first OM was asking her partner to move his finger a little bit to the left. "I realized at that moment that I had *never* told him what I wanted during sex before, and we'd been together for twenty-two years!" she said. "A little voice told me that if I could get comfortable asking for what I really want during sex, that alone could revolutionize my entire world."

The Other Side of Orgasm

That little voice of intuition was the voice that first drew me to OM. It's the same voice that brings students to my class, and I'd wager it's the same voice that has brought you this

far. I like to think of it as the voice from the other side—
the other side of *orgasm*. Because that's what we experience when we OM: a side of orgasm that is slow, deep,
and extended, rather than fast, fiery, and climactic. This
more female side has no real beginning and end. It has
multiple peaks and valleys; it is saturated and roundabout
and complex—a lot like a woman's anatomy, in fact. It is
unfathomably deep and lush with hydration. It nourishes
not the part of us that wants a smashing finale, but the part
of us that wants insight, ignition, and intimacy. The part
that wants to have richer sex—and a richer life.

Without frequent access to the kind of slow, deep orgasm
that OM offers, we're missing out on half of the nutrients
we need in life. At the risk of sounding dramatic, it's as if
all of us—men and women alike—are suffering from an
orgasmic deficiency, whose symptoms include but are not
limited to the following:

- difficulty connecting to other people
- lack of true intimacy within relationship
- deficit of sexual turn-on (especially in women)
- inability to feel sensation or be present in our own
  bodies
- disconnection from our own desires
- underlying sense that something more is possible, in
  sex and in life

Orgasm is the primary source of this nourishing, hydrat-
ing sensation we crave. Slow Sex teaches everything you
need to know to be able to access this more female side of
orgasm as frequently as you need it and as deeply as you
want to take it. The ingredients that form the foundation

of the practice of OM—stripping down, paying attention to sensation, and asking for what you desire—are the proverbial keys to the kingdom. Together they give us access to everything we've known was possible from sex: an appreciation of our own genuine experience, an unending source of turn-on, and the true intimacy we've known was possible but haven't been able to access.

Now, if that's not three good reasons to put OM on your to-do list, I don't know what would be. So let's get started, shall we?

Chapter Three

How to OM

Whenever someone asks me why I OM, the first answer that comes to mind is the simplest: OMing feels *good*. It feels connected and sensuous and nourishing and whole. It soothes, satiates, renews, and energizes. It is simply the most delicious physical experience I have ever had. When I first heard about OM, of course, it didn't sound like much. A very simple stroke, a limited time period—could it really be that big a deal? Just hearing the instructions, you can't really understand how deeply it can touch you, how quickly it can activate all of your pleasure centers, how exquisitely, deliciously precise a single stroke can feel—for the stroker and the receiver alike. You simply have to go to the kitchen and feel it yourself. So let's get cooking. Here is your primer on the steps of the practice of Orgasmic Meditation.

Step One: Asking for an OM

You can feel the whole world in a single stroke of OM. All the pleasure and the pain and the joy and the sadness that are part of our sex lives and our relationships and our lives in general—all of it can be felt in just one stroke. The same could be said of the first step of the practice: asking someone to OM with you. In the act of extending toward another person, expressing your desire, and inviting them to share such an intimate experience, you can taste everything you could ever want from the practice itself: all the enjoyment, all the connection, all the nourishment you are looking for. You let go of expectation and strategy, feel the sensations in your body, and ask for what you desire—the rest takes care of itself.

That doesn't mean it will be easy, especially at first. Even for couples who have been together for a long time (and perhaps especially for couples who have been together for a long time) it can feel very vulnerable to voice a sexual desire. The thought alone can set off a fireworks display of fears, leaving us raw and edgy in our most tender spots. If we do find the courage to ask, we then have to field the response. There are few moments as saturated with sensation as the moment a request for sex has crossed your lips and is still hanging in the air, waiting for either acceptance or rejection. We can't seem to help assigning a lot of significance to the outcome. If she says yes, it means you are attractive, acceptable, desirable, sexy. If he says no, it means you are the opposite of all those things. These are, of course, just interpretations; they are not the truth. They complicate matters, as a student of mine recently discovered. He had asked his wife for an OM one morning, and she asked if they could do it after work instead because she had an early meeting.

"That's what she said," he told me, "But what I heard was that she isn't attracted to me anymore, and she wants to postpone sex as long as possible. Since I've been OMing, I'm learning to notice where my mind goes. I saw immediately how much interpretation I was adding to what she had actually said." The key is to remember that we have a choice. We can strip down and be present for whatever answer we get, without making it more complex than it needs to be. The graceful simplicity of a "yes" or a "no" can be enough.

Luckily, there is a law of the universe written somewhere that says the more we do something, the less it has the ability to terrify us. So it is with asking for an OM. One thing that helps is to strip down the request to the bare essentials. Be as simple, direct, and honest as possible when you're asking. "Would you like to OM?" is all you need to say. You can let go of the song-and-dance routine, the romantic lines, the beating around the bush that normally come with making a sexual request, and simply ask. There is power in the clean, honest, straightforward communication of a desire. At the very least, it begs to be met by a similarly honest response.

Pay attention to the sensations in your body while you ask. We often get a whole lot of sensation when we start asking for OMs. It might begin as a sparkly explosion somewhere in your thoracic zone, contracting briefly before expanding, Big Bang–like, throughout the rest of your body. Perhaps you notice whether it starts directly at the center of your being, or if in truth it starts a little off to the left and kind of farther in back. Whether it seems to travel more up or more down; whether it stops at the tips of your tingly fingers or instead seems to expand beyond the confines of your physical body. There's something magical about simply agreeing to stay in the experience, come what may, rather than stepping even a half inch to the left or to the right. When we step out of our experience, what we tend to step into is commentary and/or interpretation. If you really commit to feeling your body, the sensation itself is so fascinating that you have little time to think about much else.

Exercise. How to Ask for an OM

- Use the question to trigger as much sensation as possible in you and your partner. Often we try to limit the amount of sensation we might cause because we're afraid we can't handle it. So we'll play it off with humor, pretend we don't care one way or the other what response we get, or make the request about need rather than desire. Resist the temptation to deaden sensation. Ask the question in the simplest but most authentic way you possibly can, and then let the sensation spread out to your whole body as you await your partner's reply.

- Feel your vulnerability. By asking for an OM, you are turning on the lights, so to speak, and admitting your own desire to be sexual. This is unfamiliar territory for most of us. Most of the time, our fear of rejection keeps us from asking openly for the connection we crave. Stepping forward with your request becomes an opportunity to feel your own soft spot, your own heart.

- Be gentle with yourself and your partner. Your desire is like a tender shoot; treat it with great kindness, as if it were someone else's precious possession that has been left in your care. Resist the temptation to demonize your partner if he or she says no, or to beat yourself up for asking. It's the offer they're turning down, not you. Let them know you honor their response, and don't be afraid to honor yourself for the courage it took to ask.

The OM itself begins the moment the date is actually set. As the anticipation builds, so does the sexual energy. Pay attention to the sensation "in the in-between," right here, right now. Conventional wisdom says that the most potent sensation can be felt at the culmination of a sensory experience—at the climax, or in this case, once the OM has begun—but you may find that you actually experience more sensation before you lie down to practice. It may come in the form of overt anticipation, turn-on, or excitement. It may also come in the disguise I call "tumescence," which is when turn-on is building in the body and gets frozen because it has no place to go. The result can be less than sexy: the urge to cry, pick a fight, call off the OM, or zone out by [insert preferred method for zoning out here].

Instead, try and stay alert. Notice what's happening inside of you. And, if you can remember, feel for your desire. It's the moments just prior to getting what we want that offer the richest experience of longing, of yearning. Don't believe me? Think back to what you felt like just before your first kiss. All that wanting, about to be realized. Try to stay that present as you move closer and closer to your OM.

"We OM a couple of times a week, at night. I started to notice I would get a little excited and aroused at work in the late afternoons. It's like I would start wanting to bounce off the walls. Then I realized it was always on the days we OMed, like something was already building. It was kind of cool when I noticed that." —Gretchen, 28

Step Two: Setting Up the Nest and Getting into Position

There is a beautiful coffee shop near where I write, where they make each cup of coffee using an individual drip filter. Each cup is brewed to order, and you get to watch them dampen the filter, grind the beans, and then pour the hot water over the grounds using a copper kettle. There is something infinitely richer about the coffee that results because you have watched them carefully tend to your particular cup. Their slow attention somehow adds a special, magical quality. It's the same magical quality that comes from carefully setting up the space where you will OM. While the OMing space or "nest" is simple, even practical, take the time to create it intentionally. Lay down blankets, place the pillows, make sure the timer is set, and then position yourselves. This slow approach is very different from the way we usually operate, especially when it comes to sex. In sex, we tend to react to a feeling of hunger by trying to feed it as quickly as possible. In the process, we miss out on feeling the sensation of our own desire. We keep our eyes on the prize of climax, never slowing down long enough to savor, appreciate, and be nourished by all the sensation that is available in the plateau that comes just prior to "going over." If we were to take this same finish-line approach in OM, we would miss out on the sensation of sexual energy, building as the space is being prepared. As we carefully retrieve everything we will need, we get to feel our own anticipation for the OM that is to come—some sweet sensation, indeed.

A different reason to take care in preparing the space is that the nest we're creating needs to feel comfortable, safe, and secure enough so that both partners can truly relax. We

72

know that the pillows will support us and that the supplies will be within reach, so there's no fear that the experience will be interrupted in the middle. We have everything we need right there. As I mentioned earlier, women especially have a physiological need to feel safe and held during sex, or we have a hard time relaxing into orgasm. Taking the time to set up a warm, cozy nest is the best way to help her ease effortlessly into the OM.

When I mention to my students that the primary responsibility for creating the nest falls to the stroker, the revelation usually results in a few raised eyebrows. From a conventional perspective OMing might already look like it is out of balance—the man almost always strokes, and the woman almost always receives. This division of labor is intentional. One of the most revolutionary benefits of OM is that it gives us the rare opportunity to reset our systems, stripping away all the ideas we have about how things are "supposed" to go, so we can sink down and experience what *is* actually happening, right now. We begin by reversing all our norms and test-driving something new in their place. This reversal may look like it caters unfairly to the women, but many men discover that there is something deep within them that gets touched—and feels inexplicably good—when they are called into service in this way.

Male Stroking

"What about the men?"

This is one of my favorite questions. Which is a good thing, since I get it all the time. The first question most people have about OM is what the practice entails; the second is, "What about the men?"

The question they're asking is whether a man ever gets the chance to be stroked—if there's any reciprocity in this picture. The answer is that yes, it is possible to stroke a man. In fact, I've included instructions in the appendix. If you're wondering why female stroking gets its own chapter while male stroking is relegated to the appendix, you're probably not alone. The fact that the practice is mostly about stroking the women goes against our sense of give-and-take, our standard sexual accounting. But unless the practice is happening between two men, I always have couples begin with female stroking exclusively. I introduce male stroking only after the couple has been practicing OM for six months or more. There are two reasons why we begin this way. First, before we can really make Slow Sex our default, we have a lot of unlearning to do. Though individual cases may vary, on the whole women tend to have a lot (and I'm talking *a lot*) of negative conditioning regarding sex. Much more than men do, in fact. Until we thaw out the iceberg of fear and shame that encases a lot of female sexuality in our culture—a thawing out that happens naturally when she is stroked—there is a tendency for her to return to her old habits of pleasing and trying to make sex look a certain way. For some women this melting happens quickly; for others it can take months or even years. Regardless of how long it takes, it's worth it in the long run to clear her system first. Once she is truly turned on, she can be a much more potent force in helping him melt his personal icebergs.

The second reason we start by stroking the women is to allow the men to explore the territory of orgasm in a new way. The orgasmic experience of OM is not the exclusive territory of the person being stroked. As the man becomes more <u>attuned</u> to his partner's body, he begins to feel a lot of sensation himself. This is a revelation to most of us, because we've always thought that orgasm could be felt only within the physical confines of the person "having" it. But that's just because we haven't honed our sensory equipment. Once we strip sex down and really pay attention to our sensations, we discover that <u>we are able to feel the orgasm happening in other people's bodies as well as our own.</u> Women, who have a natural capacity for connection, tend to get this intuitively. Men tend to need more practice in order to feel it—practice that comes, conveniently, through stroking. So as tempting as it may be to make OM a give-and-take experience, my advice is to leave the rule of reciprocity aside for now and focus exclusively on stroking her for the time being.

"I started to cry during my first OM. I couldn't believe that I didn't have to give anything in return for the attention he was giving me. It was the first time in my life."
—Elaine, 52

"At first, I was very sexually stimulated by seeing and touching her pussy. I just wanted to have sex. But after a couple of months, our OMing has become more relaxed and rhythmic. I get less aroused, and instead I've become aware of the tingling in my fingers and the swirling in my stomach. I'm more tuned into unpredictable events like a sudden loud moan from my partner, and I'm noticing the unconscious response of my body as it aligns with each new moment."
—Seth, 27

Exercise. Nesting: Setting Up for Your OM

Choose the Space. Decide on a private, comfortable location where both you and your partner can relax—a bed is probably the most intuitive choice, though some new strokers find it easier to get into position if they sit on a firmer surface, like the floor. Couples who live together also sometimes prefer to OM somewhere other than their primary bed, to differentiate their nest from the space they use to sleep and have regular sex. Wherever you choose to OM, remember to reserve the nest you create for OMing only. If you decide you'd like to have sex or even just spoon a little bit afterward, move to a different location or put the nest away first.

Set Up the Nest. A primary component of OM is the stroker's ability to see what he's doing, so the lights remain on during the OM. That said, the lighting should be soft and inviting—well-lit, but not alarmingly bright.

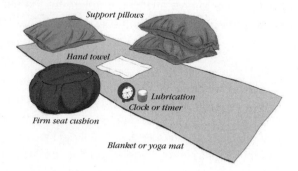

Support pillows

Hand towel

Lubrication

Clock or timer

Firm seat cushion

Blanket or yoga mat

Set up the support pillows where you will be OMing. The pillows can be arranged in a triangle: one for under her head, one for under her left knee, and one or two for the stroker to sit on. If there is any chance of her feet getting cold, consider keeping a blanket nearby. To keep things moving as smoothly as possible during the OM, you'll want a personal lubricant of some kind. (After many years of trying out different lubes, I have some favorites. See Further Resources for more information about lube or to purchase a complete OMing kit.) You'll also want a hand towel to keep the lube situation in check, and a timer—preferably one whose ring isn't too loud or abrupt. If you decide to use the timer on your cell phone, ensure that the notification sounds for incoming calls, texts, and e-mails are turned off. (Nothing like hearing your special "Mom" ringtone while you're in the middle of an OM.)

Undressing. Part of the ritual of OM is for the receiving partner to take off her clothes from the waist down, but keep the rest of her clothes on. The stroker remains fully dressed. This is one more way we differentiate OM from regular sex, and it helps keep the partners focused on the sensation of orgasm that can already be felt rising between them. There is no right or wrong way for her to undress—the simpler, the better. There is no need to add anything to the process, not even modesty. All she needs to do is to undress. No more, no less.

> "At first I was really conscious of the fact that I was taking off my pants. Like, 'here I go...taking off the pants...' but that only lasted for a couple of OMs. Then it just felt really free. It started to feel like one of the most exciting parts of the OM."
>
> —Katy, 23

Indeed, undressing is a moment to savor, for both partners. Taking off her pants and revealing herself is the moment when she truly commits to the OM. If you're the stroker, try to feel her commitment when it locks in. Taking off her clothes is the point where her "yes, in theory" becomes a "yes, we're doing this." It is a very potent moment, especially for new OMers. Taking off her clothing is an act of exposure; she is letting her partner into her personal space. The result is high sensation, even for couples who have been together for a long time. After all, it's rare for both partners to be looking with this much attention at her pussy. This fact can be confronting for both of them, as well as extraordinarily intimate. Try to be there for the sensations of both.

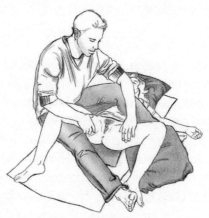

The OMing position

Assume the Position. Lay down the hand towel in the center of the nest, and guide your partner to lie down so the towel is under her rear end. The towel is a practical strategy— it keeps lube from getting all over your bed/blanket/bearskin rug.

Guide your partner to butterfly her legs open, with her left knee supported by a pillow and another pillow under her head. Her right knee will be supported by your body. When she is comfortable, sit on the pillow at her right, sliding your right leg beneath hers and putting your left leg over her belly. Position her left foot so it is resting against your right calf or foot. (Make sure her foot is not resting on *top* of your leg, or you'll experience what we lovingly call "OMing Leg"—a temporary but uncomfortable lack of sensation with death-by-pins-and-needles not far behind.)

Use as many pillows, folded blankets, and other supports as you need. Some strokers like a pillow beneath their left foot, while others want one to support their right knee. Feel free to improvise here; the goal is to find a position you can stay in for fifteen minutes with minimal adjustment. (You should, however, feel free to adjust at any time if you need to—you may need to shift around quite a bit during your first few OMs as you get used to this new position.) Many new strokers find they become tense in the neck, shoulders, and arms. Try to bring your attention to these areas and relax them consciously before the practice begins.

If you discover a variation of this posture that is more comfortable for you, by all means use it. The stroker may want to sit with his back up against a wall for support, or play with the number of pillows he's sitting on so he is higher or lower. Eventually you will find the right combination for you. One of the biggest challenges for men starting to OM is finding a posture they can hold comfortably for the duration of the OM—so if you're having a hard time, you're not alone. Keep trying different adjustments while you get used to it. Over time the position truly does become second nature.

Once you are seated comfortably, take a deep breath and feel your body. Get in touch with the sensations that are already beginning to build between you and your partner. What do you feel in your stomach? Your chest? Your genitals? Once you have made contact with what's going on inside, turn your attention back toward your partner and move into the "Noticing" step.

Step Three: Noticing

Noticing is where the stroker looks at his partner's genitals and speaks a few sentences describing what he sees. My female students tend to cringe a little bit the first time they hear about this step. He's going to gaze at *that*? And then...*talk about it*? Most women have a very different relationship with our private regions than our male counterparts. While guys have been conditioned to feel pride about their penises, we women have gotten the opposite message about our lady parts. We've been told our pussies are messy, funny-looking, and have the genital version of halitosis. Given all the judgments we've been subjected to, the thought of someone actively observing us can dredge up a lifetime of embarrassment.

The "P" Word

One reason I love OM is that it gives both men and women the opportunity to let go of any hard feelings that might exist between them and the female genitals. And sadly, if you've grown up on the grid in Western society, you most likely have a complicated relationship with the pussy. It's almost impossible to avoid. If you're a woman, then it's likely you're right this very minute having a problem with the fact that I'm using the word "pussy" at all. Why *that* word? Fact is, it's the perfect word. Vagina, genitals, the c-word-that-dare-not-speak-its-name—none have the soft, tender sensibility of "pussy." The word has grown on me, and on my students as well. Maybe it will grow on you, too—maybe not. But imagine: if we can let go of the idea that this word itself is dirty, perhaps we can also let go of the similar connotations we have for the body part it describes. (The same goes for the word "cock," whose sexiness quotient far exceeds that of "penis" or "dick." Try it: you might just find yourself wanting to use it. A lot.)

For this very reason, I remember the noticing step as the most significant moment of my own first OM. I was lying there, frozen like a Popsicle, as my partner shined a light on my genitals and started describing them. "Your inner labia look like coral. There is a deep rose color at the edges and it fades into a pearlescent pink at the base. I can see your clitoris peeking out from beneath your hood, which is tilted slightly to the side." At first I was mortified. But he went on like this for a good two or three minutes, and over the course of that time I started to soften. It was the weirdest experience I'd ever had in my life, but by the time he was, some part of me had melted. He'd given me the most precise, detailed vision of my own genitals I'd ever had. I realized that I had never really looked at my pussy. I couldn't stop the emotions from rising up. Tears streamed down my cheeks. He had looked "down there" with such clean attention. His tenderness unlocked something inside of me.

I hear similar stories from my students all the time. Heidi, one longtime OMer, talks about how difficult it was to start the practice because she disliked her genitals so much. Her self-esteem had long been so low on this front that she'd never really enjoyed receiving oral sex, for fear her partner would actually look at what he was doing.

It was a revelation, then, when an OM partner said to Heidi, after a particularly sensational session, that he thought her privates were beautiful.

"I was completely shocked and made him repeat what he'd just said," she tells me. "I couldn't believe it. Over the next few weeks I watched as my own feelings toward my pussy changed. Just having my partner's approval started to unravel a whole lifetime of my own judgments. It's amazing how quickly that can happen."

Noticing begins when you, the stroker, place your attention on what you see. Describe it using words that connote color, shape, and relative location, and try to avoid offering an interpretation of what you see. Even positive interpretations—statements about how beautiful, elegant, or otherwise fantastic her pussy looks to you—should be held for later. (Don't forget to tell her later, though!) We rarely receive feedback from other people that is not tinged with their own judgment, whether positive or negative. It can be an amazing experience during OM for a woman to simply be seen, just as she is. It is also liberating for the stroker: if you describe how you feel about what you see, what if you don't like it? (And you may not like it at first— that's not uncommon.) The temptation is to slip into white lie territory, to try to make her feel good, at the sacrifice of authenticity. So simply tell the truth of what you see—its color, shape, and relative location. Your clean attention has a much more powerful effect than any compliments you could add to it.

"Normally, when a guy talks to me about how I look, he's not saying much about me—he's talking about his opinion of me. This was the first time I felt like he was actually seeing *me*, describing *me*. It felt like I was inside of his body looking back at me, and it was amazing. I have always hated my private parts. But when he described them, I liked them for the first time. He didn't say they were pretty, and I wouldn't have believed it if he did. Just the way he described them, they sounded nice."   —Maggie, 35

"My first experience with oral sex wasn't great, and from then on I just got it in my brain that, 'this place is scary.' I didn't want to go down there, not like it, and then hurt her feelings. So instead, I would just avoid it completely. I would rather not have sex than hurt someone's feelings. Now that I've been OMing, it's night and day. I have so much more bandwidth there. The pussy has become demystified. It's gone from scary to intriguing to fascinating to *Oh my God, there is a whole thing here that's fucking amazing!*"   —Dan, 38

The Anatomy of a Woman

For both men and women, the pussy can be mysterious terrain. Many of us girls whipped out the mirrors at age twelve while reading *Our Bodies, Ourselves*, and haven't looked down there much since. Men have probably spent more time studying us, but they still seem to have a hard time finding our sweet spot. So I find that a little geography lesson is in order.

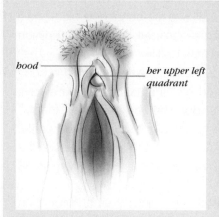

hood

her upper left quadrant

The clit

Because almost everyone knows his or her way around a penis, it can be helpful to use the analogy of a man's genitals in understanding a woman's. The exposed head of the clitoris is like the head of a man's penis. It is roughly the size and shape of a pea, although it can be significantly larger or smaller. It is highly sensitive, containing eight thousand nerve endings—double the number of nerve endings on its male counterpart and the most nerve endings in any part of the human body, full stop. In order to best see her, you may need to pull back the clitoral "hood," in the same way you would

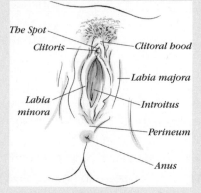

The Spot

Clitoris

Labia minora

Clitoral hood

Labia majora

Introitus

Perineum

Anus

The full female anatomy

pull back the foreskin of an uncircumcised penis. You'll notice the head of the clitoris pops out and can become enlarged with touch. Note that when we say we stroke the "upper left quadrant" of the clit during OM, we're talking about *her* left.

Just like the head of a penis, the tip of the clitoris is only the tip of the iceberg. Like the head of a man's penis, the woman's clitoris is the end of a shaft. The difference is that the shaft of a woman's clitoris runs inside of her body, just under the skin. Starting at the clitoral tip, the clitoral shaft leads back through the hood and then forks into two "crura," which extend downward along either side of the vaginal opening. In its entirety, the clitoris looks like an upside down letter Y that is bent forward at the top. The bent tip of that Y is the clitoral tip itself.

Most people think that the tip of the clit is all they have to work with, but no! Just like a guy gets pleasure from being stroked all along his shaft, a woman can experience orgasmic pleasure through stimulation of any part of the clitoris. As Masters & Johnson pointed out years ago, all female orgasms are of clitoral provenance. So-called vaginal orgasms, including orgasms that come during intercourse, come from the stimulation of the clitoral tissues.

That said, the tip of the clit is a great place to begin, thanks to the aforementioned abundance of nerve endings and its prime real estate. So it's the focus of our attention during OM.

Step Four: How to Stroke

For most people, even those of us who have been practicing for a long time, the experience of OM is hard to categorize. It's kind of like sex, because it involves arousal and sexual energy and body parts we generally encounter only in that context. But at the same time, it's also not like sex, because it is just a stroke, and it lasts only fifteen minutes, and there is no goal. There is nothing expected between the partners except attention to the stroke itself. This is where we get to put our money where our mouth is when it comes to stripping down and adding nothing extra. OM is not the time for fancy techniques or signature moves, for performance or expectation, for romance or reciprocity. The idea is not for the stroker to "make" his partner feel anything in particular. It's not about getting her to climax particularly. Instead, the stroker simply strokes his partner's clit softly, and both partners pay attention to what happens in the process.

> "After my first OM, I felt baffled—confused. It didn't feel like masturbation or sex or anything I'd ever experienced before. It didn't even feel like what it was—my boyfriend simply stroking my clitoris softly. It was something new. I wanted to scoff at it. I wanted to brush it off and explain it away. But I had to admit that something unexplainable was going on. Something great and unexpected."
>
> —Noelle, 29

When the noticing step is complete, you are ready to begin the OM. Set your timer for fifteen minutes. Safeport your partner by telling her that you are about to initiate contact. Begin by touching her legs, applying some pressure to her thighs with the palms of your hands. You might gently place a hand on her stomach to see if you can feel what she is feeling in her body. Once you feel connected to her physically, safeport her again: tell her that you are going to put your right hand into position. Slide your right hand under her buttocks, and place your thumb lightly against her vaginal opening, or introitus.

Once your right hand is in place, situate your stroking arm, beginning with resting your left elbow on your left knee. Try to maintain a straight line from your elbow to your finger without breaking at the wrist. Once your left arm is in position, you are ready to begin.

Exercise. How to Stroke a Woman

1. Place lube on your left pointer finger, and let your partner know you are about to make contact.
2. Using that same finger, stroke once upward from her vaginal opening or introitus, ending at the upper left of her clit, spreading lube over her clit as you go.
3. Using your thumb and middle finger, pull back her hood so that you can see her clit. Then place the tip of your left pointer finger on the upper left quadrant (*her* upper left) of her clit, and slide it around a bit until there is a feeling of it "locking into" her perfect spot. Finding her spot will take practice, so don't be discouraged if it takes some time before you feel confident. Ask your partner to let you know when you hit it, if that's helpful.

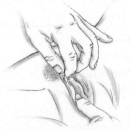

Finding her spot with his index finger

4. Begin to stroke her clit slowly, up and down, with the tip of your pointer finger. Use the lightest possible pressure to begin with, and increase from there. The strokes should be relatively short, no more than half an inch in length, and should be as consistent as you can make them.

5. Both partners pay attention to the point of contact between his finger and her clit. Notice how orgasmic sensation rises, peaks, and falls; how sometimes the sensation feels like it is going up and other times it feels like it is coming down. When your mind begins to wander, which it inevitably will, just come back to the sensation of his finger and her clit. Everything else will unfold naturally from there.

During the early stages of OMing, the stroke is cultivating the woman's ability to receive and respond to pleasure—in other words, freeing her orgasm. With every stroke old blockages start to thaw. Soon, the icebergs of shame and repression and parental disapproval and embarrassment—icebergs that are holding her desire hostage—start breaking up. Over time, they give way completely. At that point, the stroke starts filling her tank, building a foundation of sexual energy. Over time, she increases her capacity to get more and more turned on.

In other words, there is a lot more going on when you OM than meets the eye. Still, that doesn't mean it's going to *feel* like there's a lot going on—at least not at first. A lot of women have a hard time feeling the stroke at all in the early days of OM. If that's the case, don't worry; it's completely normal. I barely felt anything when I first started practicing myself. We have a lifetime of desensitization that needs reversing, and it takes more time for some of us than for others. Even once you *do* start to feel the stroke, you may or may not climax. Again, this is not a problem, either. Though individual experience may vary, climax is not a regular part of OM for most women.

> "When they said it was going to be a light stroke, I didn't know they meant *that* light. It was much lighter than I expected. I almost couldn't feel it at first."   —Katelyn, 21

With practice, a stroke that began so light and soft it was almost hard to feel becomes more and more potent. Both her genitals and his finger develop an exquisite level of sensitivity, to the point where they can feel much more than they did at the beginning—and often, much more than either would have expected. It's a matter of the body learning to relax and receive sensation. When the icebergs in the body start to break up and float away, the result is more freedom, more capacity for enjoyment, and a more sensitive sexual experience. And the more sensitive we both get, the less we need fancy moves or techniques. A simple stroke becomes more than enough.

> "I was really surprised to discover how much energy I could feel coming through my finger. I hadn't really believed it was possible."   —Brian, 26

> "Resistance came up the first time we OMed. I was terrified. You think it's going to be easy, but then you're actually there about to stroke her and you feel like a moron. You have this

male thing—you've been brought up with this male cockiness that's like, 'I'm a guy, I know what I'm doing.' And then all of a sudden to be that clueless around that body part—it hit my pride, it hit my ego, it hit my 'I can't perform' and 'I'm not a good lover.' It's so humbling. It's ancient—this idea that men are supposed to know what they're doing. Wow, it was really confronting at first."   —Erik, 41

Step Five: Communication

Communication is the next quietly groundbreaking step in OMing. I say quietly, because it's hard to believe that something as basic as sharing the sensations in our bodies or asking very simply for a change of stroke could have such a powerful effect on both partners. Undoubtedly communication ranks near the top when I ask beginning students what they were most surprised about during their first OMs.

"I had always thought talking during sex ruined the moment. I wouldn't have guessed it would feel so intimate."
          —Ryan, 37

"I'm pretty good at saying the right thing at the right time to turn him on during sex. But I didn't realize until I started OMing that all of that was just fake. I was holding back what I really wanted to say, which was 'can you please go more lightly' or 'there is this warm feeling of love pouring out of my chest right now.'"   —Leesa, 29

> "At first I thought, 'My partner and I already communicate during sex,' but then when I had to start telling him what I liked and what I wanted him to change during OM, I shut down. I didn't want to hurt his feelings. I realized I really never tell him what I want during sex at all." —Sara, 41

Through OM, we get comfortable first speaking our experience and then asking for what we desire. The immediate result is that we are able to achieve the most sensational experience possible during the session. But the true reward seems to come outside of the practice and even outside of sex in general. As we get used to speaking our genuine experience, to being honest about what we desire, we open up our interior experience to our partner. Being willing to reveal what's inside is the prerequisite for true intimacy. To give someone else a glimpse of the universe within—a place that has long been ours and ours alone—is to invite them to know you in a deeper, richer, more complete way.

As we strengthen our capacity for intimacy, we start to demystify communication as a whole. The muscles we develop during OM support our communication throughout our lives—from regular sex to friendships to working relationships to our family. One student recalls that in the first months after she started OMing, her communication style just naturally started to shift. "I stopped worrying about how what I was saying was going to be perceived and stopped being so careful about how I phrased certain things. I realized that I could just be genuine, I could be truthful. It opened a lot of things up for me."

So if not required, communication during OM is definitely encouraged. I usually don't have to press this point too much.

A silent OM can feel like crossing the Atlantic without a map. There is a lot of *I hope I'm doing this right,* on his part, and a lot of *I wish he would stroke just a little to the right,* on her part. A little conversation naturally sets things at ease, letting both partners get out of their heads and into their bodies.

> "Communication is the reason I keep OMing. It's helped me find my voice. When we OM I will ask for the stroke that I want, or I will be honest with him that I'm not paying attention anymore, or I'll make some sort of noise that I've never heard come out of my mouth before—and every time I'm surprised at how easy it was to be authentic. So then I'll get on the phone with my mother, and I'll say something to her that I never thought I could actually say. Something I've wanted to say to her for fifteen years, the one thing I didn't think I'd ever be able to talk about. And there, suddenly, we're talking about it. I attribute that to OM. So the one thing I would say to anyone who's just starting to OM is that you really *can* say whatever you want to say. Whatever it is, you can voice it. You can moan, or you can be quiet, or you can ask your partner to shift the stroke, whatever it is. You can say it." —Vanessa, 44

There are two different kinds of communication that come naturally during OM:

1. speaking your sensations
2. Yes/And communication

Speaking your sensations simply means talking about what you're feeling in your body—describing your sensory experience without judgment or interpretation. This practice may not seem like much, but it has a powerful effect: it gives us the chance, little by little, to connect more deeply with our partner by sharing things we normally keep inside. Sharing our sensations helps crack open old fears we all hold around speaking our truth and letting others really see us. Opening our interior room and letting another person inside is the act of true intimacy. So we practice just a little bit during OM by sharing something nobody would otherwise ever know: the sensations that are happening in our bodies.

There are no rules around speaking sensations except to do what feels good. Say as much or as little as you like; respond to your partner's sensations or simply absorb them in silence. When you do speak, try using words that describe texture, color, temperature, pressure, and motion. Describe "good" sensations and "bad" ones alike. Each sensation is a gift to your partner: you are inviting them to share with you what would otherwise be a completely private experience.

One of the best parts of speaking sensations is that sometimes—just sometimes—you'll discover that both of you are having some variation of the same experience, at the same time. That's always a moment: the first time you come face-to-face with the fact that there's more going on here than meets the eye.

The second communication style is what I call "Yes/And." Yes/And helps protect our partner's feelings, which can get hurt very easily in this sensitive realm of sex. Fear of hurting our partner is at the top of the list of reasons most people—women especially—feel uncomfortable asking for what we want from our partners in the first place. So we give a little spoonful of sugar before we ask for a shift in stroke by first mentioning something that feels good. "The pressure you're using feels great, thank you. Would you move a little more to the left?" or "I like the speed of the stroke, *and* I'd like to try less pressure." The stroker's role in the Yes/And scenario is to approve of his partner's request and put it into action.

The stroker should feel free to initiate communication from his end as well. He is invited to speak his sensations at any point, especially if he feels something unexpectedly powerful in his body. If he wants to make sure he is on course with the stroke, he can also ask for feedback using a version of the Yes/And question. He can offer her yes-and-no questions that start with "Would you like..." For example, "Would you like a firmer stroke?" or "Would you like me to move to the left?" These questions are simple enough that the receiver doesn't have to pull herself too far out of her orgasmic experience to answer them. They are also questions that can't go wrong for the stroker. If she says no, then by deduction he knows he's already doing a great job. If she says yes, then he has zeroed in on a way to make her feel even better. It's a win-win scenario.

Step Six: Grounding

Part of the stroker's responsibility is to watch the time and alert his partner when there are two minutes left in the OM. This time check is a gentle reminder for both partners to return their attention to the sensations they are feeling in their bodies. In other words, to make the most of the last two minutes of the session.

When the time is up, the stroker will slow his strokes and focus on stroking downward. As we'll discuss later, the direc-

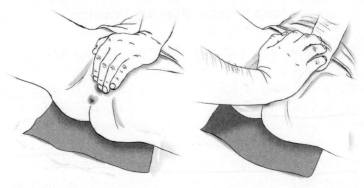

Placement of the left hand in grounding position

Both hands in grounding position

tion of the stroke makes a big difference in the flow of orgasmic energy. When you stroke your partner downward, you are beginning the process of bringing both of you back down to earth. After a few downward strokes, the stroker will continue the grounding by pressing firmly on his partner's genitals using both hands. (He might also take this opportunity to wipe off any extra lube using the hand towel.) The pressure helps stop the firing of her nerve endings, relieves the genital area of engorgement, and leaves both partners with a feeling of completion as they head back into their lives.

"Grounding to me is like taming a wild stallion. I have had OMs where we didn't ground ourselves very well when it was over, and it feels like there is all of this untamed energy flowing that makes it hard to be productive afterward. Grounding doesn't kill the turn-on that I am feeling, but it allows me to focus it and make use of it throughout the rest of the day." —Sachin, 36

Step Seven: Sharing Frames

The very last step of the OM is what we call "sharing frames." A frame is a more formal version of speaking sensations. When you share a frame with your partner, you're giving her a verbal snapshot of a particularly sensational moment you remember from the OM you just completed. There are several good reasons for sharing frames. First, putting a sensation into words helps bridge the gap between the body—which has just had a very intense experience—and the mind, which (hopefully) was in hibernation during the OM. In other words, sharing a frame helps the thinking mind comprehend what just happened to the body. Framing also seals the experience into memory. On a given day, a ton of data flies at us. We can remember only so much. OMing is one of the best things we do for ourselves—we want to lock it in. So we say the frame out loud to help remember it. If sensational moments aren't acknowledged, they tend to disappear. Sharing frames is an act of remembering—remembering that we have the capacity to be moved or awed or simply happy. In other words, why we OM in the first place.

How to Share a Frame

Just like sharing any sensation, all we do when we share a frame is report the facts of the experience. Try to stay away from value judgments like "It felt good" or "I liked it" or "I was miserable" or "I wished it would never end." Instead, drill down and talk about one particular moment, one particular sensation. Speak the details of that single sensation in terms of temperature, pressure, vibration, and experiences of spaciousness or contraction. For example:

"There was a moment when you stroked up and I felt a burst of heat in my clit that traveled up through my abdomen and radiated out through my chest."

"At one point about halfway through it was like I felt a spark of static electricity shoot out of your clit and hit the palm of my hand."

"There was a point where my whole body sort of contracted in this uncontrollable, silvery shiver."

The last reason we share frames has to do with one of the core rewards of OMing: increasing intimacy with your partner. I am always surprised when I talk to new coaching clients and discover how very little communication they have during sex. Communication *is* connection. Honest, revealing dialogue opens our interior world so that another person can actually know us deeply. Sharing frames flexes the muscle of intimacy, giving your partner a glimpse of what was going on inside you during the practice.

And as I mentioned previously, there's also the fact that more often than would be statistically expected we find that we had the same exact sensation as our partner during the OM. For those new OMers with a skeptical streak (not you, I'm sure) it can be reassuring to have evidence about what is actually happening here—even if it defies scientific measure.

OM Checklist

No matter how simple the practice seems, I find that there can be a sense of disorientation and performance anxiety during the early days of OMing. So here's a checklist to

ou focused, on track, and relaxed. Keep it handy
your early OM sessions and refer back as often as
you need to. Before you know it, OMing will start to feel like
second nature—no checklist required.

OM Checklist

Ask for the OM—Feel what it feels like in your body while
you do.

Set Up the Space—Create the OMing "nest" for yourself
and your partner. You'll want the space to be welcoming
and comfortable, not too warm and not too cool, well-lit
but not too bright. Make sure any distractions (like cell
phones) are turned off and preferably left in another
room. Gather together what you'll need:

- 3–4 pillows
- a yoga mat or heavy blanket, if practicing on the floor
- lube
- hand towel
- timer set for fifteen minutes

Positioning—The receiver lies down in the middle of the pillows and butterflies her legs open. The stroker sits to
her right. He rests his left leg over her body and slides
his right leg underneath her knees. His right hand slides
under her buttocks for support.

Noticing—The stroker places his attention on the receiver's
genitals, looking at them until he really sees them. Then
he briefly describes what he sees to the receiver, focusing on color, shape, and relative location.

Safeporting—The stroker tells his partner he is going to initiate contact. A simple "I'm going to touch you now" is perfect.

Lube Stroke—The stroker gives her a "lube stroke" with his left pointer finger, spreading lube from her introitus to her clit.

Stroking—The stroker begins a short, feather-light stroke in the upper left quadrant of her clit using the tip of his left pointer finger. He strokes either upward or downward, with more or less pressure, depending on feedback he gets from his partner and what he's feeling in his own body.

Communication—Don't forget to share sensations, request a shift in stroke, or ask your partner for feedback.

Two-Minute Warning—Stroker, let your partner know when there are two minutes left, simply by saying "two minutes."

Grounding—Once the stroker calls "time," he applies pressure to his partner's genitals using the palms of his hands. He then uses the hand towel to remove any excess lube.

Sharing Frames—The partners each share a particularly memorable moment of sensation from the OM.

Stroking for Your Own Pleasure

The early days of OM are not always easy on a stroker. We all know that sex is more complicated than it looks, and I'm afraid Slow Sex is no different. As simple as the instruction appears, fear and insecurity can and often do plague both partners, especially at the beginning. I've tried all sorts of tactics, from heavy praise to reverse psychology, in order to convince new students to believe me when I say *it's okay* and *you're doing great*. (It is, and you are—I promise!) Interestingly, the most success I've had has come when I give one little piece of advice to the stroker (within earshot, of course, of his partner). The advice is this: when in doubt, stroke for your own pleasure, rather than hers.

Strange how far a little dose of self-interest can carry you. For the guys, it seems to give permission to turn down the volume on the running commentary that says, "you aren't doing this well enough." It takes his focus off watching her for signs of get-off (and then launching into self-recrimination if she doesn't seem to be experiencing the "appropriate" level of enjoyment) and instead turns the focus inward. How does *he* feel in his body when he strokes up? When he strokes down? When he applies more pressure, or less? How can he draw pleasure of his very own from every stroke he makes? This tiny shift in focus has been known to result in a sea change in terms of his experience. Suddenly strokers find themselves flooded with greater sensation than they ever thought would be possible from any activity, not to mention one where their pants are still on.

> "If my partner is only trying to 'give' pleasure while stroking, it feels like someone is trying to 'do' something to me. This is not nearly as pleasurable for me as when he is stroking as much for his pleasure as for mine. I think it has to do with how attentive he's being to the sensation while OMing. It's the same way that you can tell if someone enjoyed making a meal or if they just threw it together. One wants to be savored, the other consumed."
>
> —Diana, 45

Interestingly, receivers value this instruction just as much as their strokers. <u>When she knows he's focusing on his own pleasure, it takes some of the pressure off</u>. Performance anxiety can be a big part of a receiver's early OM practice. We women may be tempted to default to old habits of augmenting our experience, attempting to reassure him that he's doing well by turning up the volume—breathing, moaning, and moving in ways that may not be entirely genuine. Knowing that he's supposed to be stroking for his own pleasure makes it easier to strip down and focus on bare sensation—nothing added.

Of course, all this takes practice. Nobody gets their first OM "just right." Some are blown away in orgasmic bliss, others are not. But I have never encountered a couple who didn't discover something new, unexpected, and extraordinary. After your first OMing session you may not quite understand what you just experienced, but if you're anything like my students you will know it was like nothing you've ever done before.

You will probably also have questions—lots of them. So before we do anything else, let me open the floor to some Q&A. You should find the answers to most of the questions you have in the next chapter, Troubleshooting.

Chapter Four

Troubleshooting

When people ask me why I chose to become a sex teacher, I like to lean in and whisper, "The orgasm made me do it!" In truth, I'm only half joking. It was indeed the feeling I had when I OMed for the first time that changed everything, that altered the entire course of my life and sent me down the long and winding path that has led me to where I now stand. First and foremost, it told me that the plans I had at the time to enter the San Francisco Zen Center were not going to work; how could I become a monastic after what I'd just experienced? Not that I *knew* what I'd just experienced. I knew the event was going to alter my life in some way, far more than I could even have imagined at the time. I knew this new version of orgasm had already reset my compass. I knew I needed to be heading toward more of *that* feeling...

But what *was* that feeling? It was kind of like climax, but it wasn't. It was kind of a spiritual experience, but not exactly. How was I supposed to be heading toward it for the rest of my life if I couldn't even define it?

My mind couldn't figure it out, but my body knew. This same sweet disorientation floods the room when my students return from their first OM session. It's like they've ripened in that fifteen minutes; they are open and soft. That's not to say they're all floating on a cloud of orgasmic bliss—some of the guys are holding their lower backs awkwardly, wondering what to make of that position. Some of the women have their hands in the air already, prepared to make the case that the stroke should be firmer, longer, and/or in a different location.

There is not a pale face in the room, however. Everyone seems to be illuminated from within, their rosy cheeks and bright eyes confirming that something entirely new has just happened. And I recognize it, because it's the same thing that happened to me all those years ago.

Unfortunately, since I am technically the sex teacher, they want me to explain it to them.

"It was just his finger on my clit…why was it so different?"

"Where does that…electricity…come from?"

"Just tell us," they're all pleading, "what *was* it?"

The problem is, even after all these years, even after teaching this to hundreds of students, I still don't know how to answer that question. All I know is that it's something, and that getting to teach this "something" is way more fun than being in a Zen monastery.

Luckily for me, swiftly on the heels of wonder comes a stampede of logistical questions, and those I can answer just fine. You may be having some of these questions, too. So let me share them with you here: some of the frequently asked, *answerable* questions—first for her, then for him, and finally for both of them together.

Troubleshooting for Her

I didn't have a climax. Is that okay? I put this one first because no matter what you call it, if it has "sex" in the title, we assume it must be about climax. For many women, the question of climax has been bubbling on the back burner for years, and OM only turns up the flame. It is not just that they want climax—although they do—it's that they want to know that they are not broken. They want to know that they are not missing some vital capacity that comes to other women, and apparently most men, with effortless ease. They fear that lack of climax equates to sexual ineptitude, and the fact that they didn't climax during their first OM has once again demonstrated their deficiency.

So here are the facts: many women do *not* climax, or "go over," during OM. This isn't to say that it's verboten or wrong or a problem if you *do* end up climaxing during the session— some women certainly do. But it's sort of neither here nor there. The goal of the practice, if there is one, is simply to feel the stroke and the sensation it generates. You're learning how to apply attention to the feeling of orgasmic energy in the body. As a result, you have the chance to really feel your own sexual desire in a way few of us have the opportunity to do. As for the fear of feeling frustrated for lack of a climax, the second to last step of the practice—grounding—is designed specifically to reintegrate the sexual energy that has built up throughout the OM so "sexual frustration" is not a problem. "I got so turned on during the OM that I was worried when he said 'two minutes' and I hadn't come," a new student told me recently. "I was afraid I would end up feeling incomplete and horny for the rest of the day. But when he grounded me, it was like magic. I still felt turned on, but the whole thing felt complete at the same time. It was like he packed me up and sent me on my way." If your partner really takes the time to ground you, you'll leave the session feeling alive, almost electrified with sexual energy—and not at all frustrated.

Speaking of sexual energy, many women actually report that they prefer *not* to go over during OM, because they come to enjoy the way OMing *sans* climax increases their sexual energy. Whereas traditional sex is about expiating or getting rid of "excess" energy through climax, OM is a way we can *build* energy. It's an understatement to say that most women today don't know what it feels like to have a reservoir of energy we can pull from at any time. We feel like we're always hanging on by a thread. We are putting so much energy into our kids, our families, and our jobs that we don't have much left over at the end of the day. Sex often feels like just one more energy-suck. In this way OM can be a revelation: You mean I can actually use sex to *generate* energy? I can use it to increase my capacity? The answer is a big, enthusiastic YES. OM gives us the opportunity to refill our tank. The energy we get from it can then be used to nourish our everyday experience—to hydrate us so that everything we do is suffused with pleasure, from work to yoga to, yes, sex.

> "Before we started OMing I was always avoiding sex because it just felt like work. But something has changed, and now I see how integral sex is to our relationship. It is something I want to do, rather than something I feel like I have to do."
> —Tara, 35

I couldn't concentrate because I hated that he was looking...you know, down there. You'd be surprised what a big issue this is for a whole lot of women. As previously discussed, OM can bring up a lifetime of shame and embarrassment about our genitals. The good news is, it can also *heal* a lifetime of shame and embarrassment about our genitals. Many new students report that the experience of being looked at without judgment by their partner is itself as life-changing as anything the stroking itself can do. Meantime, if you're having a lot of resistance to the idea of being observed that closely, try one or both of these tips to help overcome the aversion to having your vagina on view:

- **Go get a bikini wax.** Please don't mistake my meaning here: there is absolutely nothing wrong with the natural look. The emphasis in "go get a bikini wax" is on the "go get one" part. What you'll discover, as you lie there on the table on full display, is just how totally unremarkable your pussy will be to the woman who is waxing you. The discovery that, to some people, a pussy is a pussy, was a revelation to me. Waxing professionals have seen hundreds just like yours. Yours is no less beautiful, no more weird-looking, no uglier, no less worthy of a good hard gaze than anybody else's. Regardless of the subtle social cues telling us to keep ours hidden, just one wax job and you'll discover that, to at least one person in the world, your genitalia are no big deal.
- **When in doubt, name your fear.** Talk to your partner about your concerns. There's something about communication that has the power to crack even the most intractable fear. We're not trying to guilt-trip him into proclaiming your parts the prettiest he's ever seen— though he might say just that. No, the point has more

to do with you than with him. Just like naming your sensations, naming your fear has a magical effect. Sometimes the fear dissolves on contact, like pouring water on the Wicked Witch of the West. In other cases the fear will still be there, but something about admitting it out loud gives you a better sense of what you're up against. To tame your fear, name your fear, as they say.

I couldn't feel anything. When I first started OMing, my sessions always started the same way. My partner would tell me he was going to put his finger on my clit—and then I would wait. Wait to feel his finger, wait to feel his stroke. I would wait and wait…and wait. Fifteen minutes later the only frame I would be able to offer was a careful description of what numbness feels like. After a lifetime of going harder in order to get more sensation—and yes, years of using a vibrator—my body was addicted to pressure. Without it, I couldn't feel anything.

It took—and it's embarrassing to even admit this— almost *three years* before the warm light of attention started breaking up the icebergs in my body and I could start to feel again. Quite literally, it took me longer to thaw out than anybody I have ever worked with. So if you're having a hard time figuring out what all this talk of "feeling sensation" is about, don't worry. You're not alone! After a lifetime of turning up the volume—in terms of pressure and speed—to get more sensation, most of us are just not calibrated to register a stroke that is light and slow. The good news is that in this case, practice makes perfect. Over time, and with the application of pure clean attention to the feeling of his finger meeting our clit, our bodies start to

thaw. We start to soften; we start to feel. A few OMs from
now you can expect to see some cracks forming, then big
chunks of ice floating away. Things are loosening up, and
soon a little glimmer of sensation can get through. Maybe
it's just a stroke—just one little stroke—but the sensation is
yours. Your attention and your desire have coaxed it out of
hiding, and now you know that it's possible.

So I always give new students the instruction to try to
feel one stroke—just one single stroke—during a session.
If you can feel one, the rest will come in time. Even for
advanced practitioners, the point of an OM is to really be
able to feel one stroke; just one. Everything else is icing on
the cake.

In the meantime, try this:

- **Focus on what you _do_ feel**. As I discovered in my early
  days, numbness is also a sensation. How would you
  describe it?
- **Name one thing—just one thing—you can feel**. A tickling? A feeling of heat? Some motion? Feeling anything
  at all is success here, and communicating that feeling
  only magnifies it.
- **Pay attention to your genitals**. If thoughts of failure or
  performance anxiety enter your mind, keep bringing
  your attention right back to your clit. That's the only
  thing you have to do here: lie back, relax, and keep
  your attention on the point of contact between his
  finger and your clit. There is no right or wrong experience in OM.
- **Ask for more pressure**. Though we don't want to
  become reliant on heavy pressure, it can sometimes
  help to ask your partner to increase pressure until you

_do_ feel it—then to back off slowly. Notice the point where you go from sensation to numbness again. That's the edge you're working with; over time you'll start to see that edge arriving at lower and lower levels of pressure, I promise.

- **Talk to your partner.** It's possible he's having a hard time finding just the right spot; help the poor guy! Try the Clitoral Mapping OM (see page 138), and note where around your clit you have the most sensation.

- **Give yourself a break.** Every OM, and every OMer, is different. Some sessions you can expect to feel incredible sensation, while during others you won't feel very much at all. There is no "perfect" here—inconsistency is part of the deal. See if you can find something to enjoy in every OM. Maybe it's the feeling of being held and taken care of by your partner. Maybe it's the experience of having your genitals looked at without judgment. Find just one point of pleasure you can name, and you'll have succeeded.

Oh, I felt something. It's called pain. The clit is the most sensitive spot on the female body. Although we'd love to think that its eight thousand nerve endings only pick up on the feeling of pleasure, the fact is in some cases they also pick up on pain.

Oversensitivity is something many women feel at some point during their OMing practice, especially at the beginning. Some of us are simply more sensitive than others. A direct stroke on our clit can be exquisitely pleasurable for some of us; however, for others it can send every nerve in our body jangling like a fire alarm. Women who experience the stroke as painful have equated it to the feeling of broken glass being stroked into them, or the point of a very sharp knife being driven into the clit—in other words, nothing you'd ever want to feel again. And yet many women who have had pain in their OMing continue to practice. One of our core Slow Sex teachers has had the experience of pain as part of her practice for years. What it taught her was a lesson she needed to learn in life, as well as sex. "I used to think the pain meant there was something wrong with me. I would be afraid to ask my partner to lighten up," she says. "But the pain was so intense that I finally didn't have a choice. To my surprise, he was really grateful when I asked him to adjust. I saw that he really wanted to please me, much more than I ever realized."

While for some people pain is physiological—some of us are just built with more highly sensitive clits than others—I've also heard students report pain they later believed was psychological. One student recently related some unexpected pain during practice. "Everything had been going fine for weeks, but then one day during OM it was just like he was rubbing gravel into my clit. I thought, 'What is going on here?' I asked him to change his stroke and it got better, but I still wondered. I put my attention back to the stroke, and suddenly this anger started to come up. When I looked at it more closely, I realized I was still mad about something he'd e-mailed me a few days earlier. It really wasn't a big deal, but I hadn't communicated to him that his comment had hurt me a little bit. After the OM I asked him if we could talk, and I let him in on what was going on. It was a really intimate moment. When we OMed again, the pain was gone."

Some students go further and report that pain seems to signal some sort of psychic knot that needs to be worked out. If they stay with the pain, as a sort of research project, there's often a breakthrough on the other side. This is not to say that you *should* power through your pain. Take care of yourself; take a break from OMing for a day or two, or ask your partner to change stroke—whatever you need. OMing is about enjoyment, after all. But at the same time, clit pain does not need to be a reason to stop OMing. Here are some common remedies for working with pain:

- Ask your partner to stroke more lightly and/or more slowly, until the pain subsides.
- Request that he start off the session by stroking on top of the clitoral hood instead of stroking the clit itself. As the orgasm starts to build, you can ask him to slowly move underneath the hood, if you desire.
- If any sort of motion feels too painful, ask your partner to place his finger lightly on the clit and keep it there. Then, once you feel comfortable, you can ask him to start stroking again very slowly. Feel free to ask him to return to stillness at any time, however.
- Ask your partner to stroke the lube, rather than stroking your clit itself. This can be a sensational way to practice at any time, but it's especially helpful if the clit is painful or sensitive. The stroker places a dollop of lube directly on the clit, and then strokes the lube itself gently without making direct contact with your clit.
- Inquire internally about the source of the pain. Is there anything unsaid between you and your partner? Is there any reason you might be resisting practice today?
- Be gentle with yourself. Pain can be a natural part of the OMing process for some women—*there is nothing wrong with you.* Take this as an opportunity to

practice asking your partner to give you what you need and desire. Contacting our own desire is one of the primary goals of the practice; see where it wants to take you.

I have past sexual trauma. Should I OM? This is an extremely sensitive, very personal question. And given how many women have experienced sexual trauma or abuse over the course of their lives, it's also very common—as you can imagine, it comes up a lot during our beginner Slow Sex workshops. My first recommendation to anyone who is working with sexual trauma is to see a licensed therapist or psychologist who has been trained to help in that area specifically. At the same time, many women who find their way to OM have already spent time in traditional therapy and are looking for a more experiential way to heal. For these women, I can only say that many have found peace and rebirth through this practice. Many students report that the structured nature of OM offers a sense of relaxation not usually found in more open-ended, conventional sex. You know exactly what to expect from OM: it's only fifteen minutes per session, and it's only a stroke. There is no pressure to climax or please your partner along the way—all you have to do is pay attention to your own sensation. That's not to say that OMing may not stir up difficult emotions and memories, however. If you find yourself facing painful issues during OM, here are some guidelines to keep in mind:

- Remember that you have the power to end the OM at any time. If uncomfortable feelings or memories of trauma arise during the session, communicate with your partner. Feel free to ask him to slow down or stop altogether.

- Allow yourself to feel and express any emotion you are having. As OM thaws out our blocked systems, powerful emotions of all sorts can come through. The practice is slow and deliberate enough that we find we can't railroad past our emotions the way we are sometimes able to do during sex. For this reason, many women report crying through their first several months of OM, as they allow themselves to feel sensations—both physical and psychological—that they have not felt in a very long time. You are not alone; it's part of the process and it can be incredibly sweet to let it all out. Let your partner hold the space while you allow the emotion to flow.

- Go all the way to your edge, but don't go over it. Take the time to get to know your own limitations. With each OM, be willing to nestle right up against it—but don't go past it. There is a sweet spot there, just at the edge. Be willing to taste it.

- Stay in communication with your partner throughout the OM. Let him know what sensations you're feeling, be they emotional or physical. And again, be gentle with yourself. This work requires a certain level of courage from all of us; acknowledge that it isn't always going to be easy, and take it slow.

Won't it make sex less special if we practice OM every day? This is a question that comes up at pretty much every Slow Sex workshop—but only from the women. (This thought would literally never cross a man's mind.) For women, everything is connected. When a man enters our body, he enters our heart and our head and our spirit at the same time. Because of this, sex has become, to us, a Very Big Thing. The idea of experiencing orgasm just as it is—minus the romance, the eye-gazing, the seriousness that have become prerequisites to our idea of "good sex"—is hard for women to understand at first.

As a result, we keep orgasm hidden away in the cabinet most of the time, because it's *special*. We think we are doing ourselves a favor, that by withholding the delicious sensation of sex we are somehow intensifying the pleasure received when we *do* have it. This goes back to the conditioning we've gotten about keeping our hunger at bay. If we enjoyed orgasm every single day, what might become of us? At the very least, we'll stop enjoying it so much! The same argument can apply to eating chocolate, or spending a little extra to buy flowers for our desk, or setting aside time to do something we love every day.

The assumption we're making is that if we trot orgasm out every day, over time its specialness will diminish. But in my experience, this assumption is false. One thing we learn when we start OMing is that the more awareness we place on something, the more beauty we can see in it. What we get into relationship with reveals its secrets to us. Let sex come out to play, get to know it a little more every day, and I promise you: the sensation will increase, not lessen.

> "The more we OM, the more I can feel my orgasm opening up. I had no idea how much power was inside of me."
> —Kristie, 28

Troubleshooting for Him

So…when do I get stroked? Guys, if you're finding yourselves wondering why you would ever want to spend fifteen minutes stroking your partners and getting nothing in return, then you have, as they say, arrived. Whether he admits it or not, every new stroker has asked himself at some point whether he's a Grade-A sucker for agreeing to do something so ludicrously one-sided as OM. And it's not just the guys who notice this inequity. Around hour two of the Slow Sex workshop the question of "what's in it for him?" starts bubbling up… from the *women*. Yes, the women start to raise hell on the men's behalf, wondering how they themselves are supposed to enjoy the bounty of OM with the knowledge that you guys are practically wasting away from sexual starvation.

I have never come up with a better answer to this question than this: start stroking, and see what happens. It goes against all of our preconceptions about sex and relationship, but to hear them tell it, the stroker experiences just as much orgasm during OM as the receiver does. Don't believe me? Take it from one of my students, Jennifer, half of a lesbian couple. When they first started OMing, Jennifer received and her partner stroked. Later on, they decided to switch positions.

"When we first took the workshop and decided she'd be stroking me, I have to admit I thought I was getting the better end of the deal," Jennifer says. "In the workshop the teacher said the strokers would feel just as much orgasm as the receivers, but I didn't understand how that could be.

"A few months later I decided I wanted her to have the experience of being stroked, too, so I told her I wanted to switch positions for a while. I was doing it entirely for her. It was basically an altruistic move. But the minute my finger hit her clit, it was like my finger was a valve and the orgasm just came right through it and filled up my entire body. I felt exactly the same sensation as when I was getting stroked, except it wasn't just concentrated in my genitals. It was like I was getting hit by a warm wave. I had to really concentrate to keep stroking because all I wanted to do was to feel the orgasm."

Now if that sounds far-fetched (and it does to many men, right up until they experience it for themselves), then consider some other reasons you might practice. It might be the fact that the <u>attention you develop can be transferred into every aspect of your life and relation</u>ship. Maybe it's the confidence and satisfaction that comes with knowing you're getting your woman off every time you stroke. Maybe it's that <u>stroking increases her sexual appetite</u>—which is what most women report—so you're getting a more turned-on partner in the bedroom. Who knows? All I can say is that the men (and female strokers) seem to keep coming back to this "boring" practice that's "all about her," so there must be something more here than meets the eye.

That was harder than I thought it was going to be, and I couldn't tell if I was doing it right. Once the guys are on board to start the practice, the first question that comes up is how do they know if they're doing it right. When it comes to "real" sex, the cues a man uses to know if he's pleasing his partner are primarily visual (he can see her moving in a sexy way) and audible (he can hear her moaning, breathing heavily, and even telling him how good it feels).

Just for the record, these are the easiest cues for a woman to, shall we say, elaborate on.

And—at first, anyway—neither of these particularly applies

during OM. During OM, her only instruction is to feel the stroke; to feel how orgasm is expressing itself in her body. There is no call to perform and no requirement to reassure her stroker that he's doing it right through auditory or visual cues. All she's doing is feeling. For her, this can be a freeing experience.

For him, it can feel like someone just turned off all the lights.

So the instruction I give new strokers is: keep your attention on your partner's genitals and watch for signs of orgasm there. Are her labia swelling and getting darker? Is her pussy more lubricated? Can you see her genitals contracting or vibrating? These are all signs that "you're doing it right." More obvious cues will develop over time—as her orgasm starts to open up, you can expect her to start breathing more heavily and even starting to moan with pleasure. But even if her get-off isn't audible, you don't need to worry. Sometimes the most powerful orgasm is totally silent. In fact, one of the ways to access the deepest possible orgasmic sensation is to quiet both the body and the voice.

Over time, the idea is for the stroker to start feeling, via the sensations in his own body, whether the orgasm is ignited between them. Men who have been stroking for a long time report feelings of electricity when the finger meets the clit, the sensation of warm liquid flowing throughout their own bodies, a tingly feeling from head to toe, and, of course, sexual turn-on in their genitals. All of these—and many more feelings—can be signs that things are going just as they are supposed to. But don't fret if you aren't able to feel very much in your own body at the start. This is a learning process. The more you OM, the more sensation you can expect to get.

117

And when all else fails (or even if it doesn't), there's your old standby: communication. Ask your partner yes-or-no questions about direction, speed, and pressure. Let her guide you toward what feels good for her. You'll be surprised how often the result is that you, yourself, start to feel good, too. Just remember, this whole enterprise is a process of trial and error. It's about the connection itself. As long as you feel even one stroke you give her, you're on the right track.

I couldn't find her spot. (Or: I found her spot, but then it disappeared.) On most women, the spot you're looking for is that tiny upper-left quadrant of her clit. (Though of course, as nature may have it, each woman is different. Don't worry: the Clitoral Mapping OM in the next chapter will help you find it, wherever it's hiding.) There's so much power at that one little point that many strokers find they actually feel some sort of "click" or "landing" when they touch in on it. Yep, we're back there—to intuition. In this case, you're letting the clit tell you where it wants to be stroked. Feeling for such subtle sensation takes practice, though, so don't be surprised if you have some trouble at first. The good news is that most women report getting stroked is pleasurable even if the guy doesn't quite hit her spot, and most strokers eventually get there. One new OMer describes his partner's spot as a "finger magnet"—it's as if the spot itself draws his finger in. My best advice is to let go of expectation and feel your way. But if you would feel better having some instruction, this is what I have to offer you:

- **Look closely.** Pull her hood back and see if you can locate her clit visually. It often looks like a little round bump, brighter pink than the skin around it. If you are able to see it, you'll have a better idea where to put your finger as you feel for the spot. In this case, two senses may be better than one.

- **Start slowly.** Take some time to run your finger across and around her clit, feeling for the spot before locking in. Finding the spot is an art form, so let her body speak to you through your felt sensations.

- **Try, try again.** If you found the spot and then lost it, pull back her clitoral hood and try again. It's completely normal and expected for her clit to retract at times throughout the OM, so don't sweat it. Just put your finger back into the "pocket" of her hood and feel for it again.

- **Stroke lightly.** One student says this maneuver is like "enticing the cat out from under the bed with a bowl of milk." Sometimes if you lighten your stroke, the clit will actually come out to meet you. It happens: as her arousal ignites and her genitals start to swell, her clit will often rise up and meet your finger without any effort on your part.

- **Ask for feedback.** Let your partner guide you to where it feels good. Unless she's having a hard time feeling her clit—which can be the case early on, as described previously—she will be able to tell you if you're getting warmer or not. Be sure to pose your questions in yes-or-no format ("Would you like me to move a little to the left?") so she can answer them easily while staying connected to her own experience.

I'm afraid of hurting her. Men have been conditioned to see women as delicate—especially where our private parts are concerned. And it's true, our clit can be sensitive, and sensitivity can sometimes roll over into pain. But to those men who come to our Slow Sex workshops worried they will be like a bull in a china shop down there, I have only one thing to say.

We push babies out of those things.

Okay? There's pretty much nothing you can do with the tip of your finger that's going to cause permanent damage. Even if she's feeling painfully sensitive that day, one stroke isn't going to kill her—she'll just ask you to stroke more lightly and that will be that. Still worried? There are two rather eye-opening exercises I love to give apprehensive strokers. The first one uses the moves we learned in the "grounding" step of the OM practice. With your partner's consent, press your hands firmly against her genitals as if you were grounding her after an OM. As you press, ask her if she can take more pressure. If she says yes, press harder. Continue in this way until she says that she has reached the limit of pressure she can take. You may discover that your arms give out before her pussy does.

The second practice I love for this purpose is to take hold of your partner's inner labia and pull on them gently. Slowly begin to pull more firmly, asking your partner to tell you at what point she feels the first twinge of discomfort. In almost every case I've seen, the strokers have been shocked to discover just how long it takes for her to feel the first twinge of pain. We're more resilient than we look!

The lube was out of control. It's true: it takes some practice to keep the lube where you want it—and *only* where you want it. The problem is not just one of neatness; too much lube in the wrong places and a stroker will find he is hard-pressed to keep her hood back far enough for her clit to emerge. The secret of mastering the lube is twofold: First, be judicious. Start with a small dollop and increase from there if necessary. You can always go back for more mid-OM if required. Second, make sure that when you first give her the "lube stroke," you apply the lube from the vaginal opening up to her clit, but not beyond. (See the figures on page 84 for a refresher.) Try to avoid applying it *above* the clit, on the clitoral hood itself, or you'll have a hard time keeping a steady hand as you pull the hood back to stroke.

Finally, it never hurts to keep an extra towel on hand just in case you need to wipe her down and start over. No shame there, man. No shame at all.

Sitting in that position for fifteen minutes is really uncomfortable. Unless you're a practiced yogi, the stroking posture will likely take some getting used to. The good news is that it gets easier every time you do it. In the meantime, here's a refresher on how to make the posture as comfortable as possible:

- Make sure you're well supported—your knees are supported and your back is straight. At first it can be helpful to bring several extra pillows to the OMing nest so you can adjust your posture during the OM if necessary.
- Consider OMing with your back against a wall. Some strokers find the posture more comfortable if they have something to lean against.
- Rest the elbow of your stroking hand on your left knee, and try not to break at the wrist. Both of these maneuvers will prevent arm fatigue.

- Make sure her legs aren't resting on top of your right leg. If there is any pressure at all on that leg, you have a good chance of losing the use of it for several minutes after the OM is complete.
- Throughout the OM, pay attention to what you are feeling in your upper back, shoulders, and arms. New strokers tend to focus so intently on the stroke that they don't realize their own bodies are frozen. So check in with yourself. If you're feeling tense, rigid, or stiff, take a deep breath and relax.
- If the position is so uncomfortable you can't concentrate, don't hesitate to interrupt the OM to adjust your position. Better to take a break than be miserable for the entire fifteen minutes.

I have no skills with my left hand. This is something we hear a lot from right-handed OMers, especially in the beginning. The instruction to use the left hand is entirely practical: you're stroking the upper-left quadrant of her clit, and it's simply easier to reach if you're sitting to her right and stroking with your left hand. Don't worry if it feels a little awkward at first; like the posture, it's one of those things you'll get used to in time.

She seemed to like that a little too much. I'm afraid she's never going to want to have sex again. This is a concern we hear often, and for good reason. If you're like most men, you're probably working with a sense of scarcity around the amount of sex you're having. It's natural to worry that if you turn over some of your pussy exposure time to a practice like OM, you'll end up with even less sex than you were already getting.

Here's perhaps the best news you've heard yet about OM: for most women, the experience of filling up with sexual energy during OM actually *increases* desire for "traditional" sex. In most cases, the level of turn-on women have access to when they are stroked slowly and deliberately far exceeds the amount of turn-on they get from penetration (which doesn't focus on the most sensitive spot, the upper left quadrant of her clit) or even oral sex (where we often feel torn between the experience of pleasure and the pressure to perform). So no matter how long you've been with your woman, you're very likely about to see her more turned on than you ever have before. And for most women, the result of more turn-on is an increased sexual appetite. As one longtime stroker tells it, "I had never met a woman who wanted to have sex more often than I did until I started dating in the OM community. We used to have this saying about the community that still stands: 'OneTaste. Where the women are turned on...and the men are exhausted.'"

I got hard. Sorry, it's the truth. At some point during their OMing practice, most men have had the experience of getting a hard-on. I hear that the frequency decreases the more OMing you do, however. Many men also report that the "grounding" step at the end of the OM works as well to reintegrate his sexual energy as it does to reintegrate hers. My theory is that this happens out of intention. When you decide to OM, you're agreeing at the outset to have a fifteen-minute experience with your partner. There's really no way of telling what will happen during that fifteen-minute period—you're pretty much just along for the ride—but there is one thing you can be sure of: the experience will have a "hard stop" fifteen minutes later.

So it's as if your body prepares for that inevitability even before it begins. Somehow, if you take the time to ground her well, you, too, will feel like you've had a complete experience when the OM is over.

> "I admit I agreed to go to the class because I thought OM would be a way to have sex more often. I figured her pants are going to be off, right? I thought we'd jump right into it after the stroking was over, but that wasn't the way it happened. There was something about the ritual, the grounding and the frames, that I ended up really liking. It was a really intimate experience by itself." —Ross, 43

Troubleshooting for Both

We were rocking out. It seemed a shame to end after just fifteen minutes! In our "more is better" world, it is logical to jump to the conclusion that if a fifteen-minute OM is good, then a twenty- or thirty-five- or sixty-minute OM must be better. Alas, all the rules of the regular world seem to break down in the world of OM, including this one. It's not that you *can't* go longer; it's just that you may discover you're getting a different experience than you bargained for. One of the things we're learning when we OM is how to sustain a high level of sensation for longer than a split second without automatically tamping it out. There is a lot of sensation during an OM, for both partners, and most beginning practitioners discover that fifteen minutes is long enough (and then some).

If you and your partner would like to play around with a longer session, however, I would suggest one rule: decide at the outset exactly how long you plan to OM, and then don't go over that time limit. Keeping a firm "container" of time for your practice allows both partners to really relax into the experience, knowing it has a set end point. At the same time, make sure both partners have permission to stop the OM at any time if it is getting too intense.

Should we have sex less often if we're OMing? Absolutely not. You should have as much sex as you like, in whatever positions you like, as often as you like.

I don't have a partner. Can I do this alone? The short answer is no. Although it's certainly possible to masturbate in an OM-like way for fifteen minutes, it is not the same as Orgasmic Meditation. First, OM is designed to give your voluntary mind a break—in other words, to take you out of control for a period of time. (Out of control is where we all secretly long to be. Don't take it from me.) Stroking yourself pretty much defeats that purpose. If the sensation is high, you can turn it down. If it's low, you can kick it up a notch. It's kind of like trying to tickle yourself. You may feel tickly sensations, but you're not at their mercy because you're the one doing the tickling. Same goes for OM.

The second difference between masturbation and OM has to do with the resonance that grows between the partners who are OMing. While it defies logic, when we connect deeply with another person, we create an entirely new experience between us. Our partner draws out our sexual energy, and we draw out theirs. Together, the two of us create a third thing between us—the orgasm—and

we explore it together. So while you can certainly generate pleasurable sensation by stroking yourself, you are not
practicing Orgasmic Meditation until you are plugged into
the experience with another person.

So what to do if you find yourself sans partner and
wanting to practice? As hard as it may be to believe, this is
a good, juicy place to be. Like any obstacle that might be
getting in the way of your practice, not having a partner
gives you the chance to really experience your desire to
OM. It also gives you the opportunity to extend beyond
your comfort zone, beyond your fear of rejection or shame
about wanting to do a sexuality practice—and to just ask
someone.

Yes, just ask.

The thought can send shivers of terror, I realize. *Ask*
someone? Who, a friend? Your ex-boyfriend? The barista
you flirt with every morning while she makes your latte? I
get it. A lot comes up when you consider asking someone
to OM. First, the fact that they will likely have no idea what
you're talking about, and you'll have to explain this unusual
practice in detail, on the spot. Second, that they might reject
the offer—and you, yourself, will feel rejected in the process. Third, there's the shame factor that comes with asking for what we desire sexually. The good news is that, as
discussed in the previous chapter, asking gets exponentially
easier the more you do it. Ladies, I have never met a straight
man who wouldn't be thrilled beyond recognition for you
to ask him to stroke your pussy. He might not be free to
do so, for a variety of reasons (including fears of his own),
but you can guarantee you're going to make his day just by
asking. If he declines, consider it a charitable contribution
(alas, no tax deduction available) and move on.

Guys, your situation is trickier. To be blunt, thanks to a lot of social conditioning there is a distinct possibility that you will look like a perv for asking a woman to OM. But that doesn't mean you shouldn't do so—you just need to do it very cleanly. Make the request specific; explain that it's a meditative practice rather than straightforward sex and that the goal is simply to give her a safe place to have an orgasmic experience. Emphasize that no reciprocation will be expected, nor will any such offers be accepted. (And then make sure you maintain that boundary. I suggest a forty-eight-hour hold on any offers for reciprocation she might make, to be certain her offer is coming from true desire and not because she thinks she "should" give you something in return.)

Still sound unapproachably edgy to ask someone who is not your partner to engage in a sex practice? No worries. If OMing is something you truly want to do, the obstacle of finding a partner will take care of itself. Go your own pace. Keep reading, keep thinking about it, and if you have the desire, a partner will come.

Sex isn't a problem for me—I'm not even sure why my partner dragged me here. As I said at the beginning, most students come to our Slow Sex workshops to improve their sex lives. The guys want to know how to please their women. They want to learn more about her anatomy, what brings her pleasure and what doesn't, and they want a foolproof way to get her off. The women come primarily because they want to *enjoy* sex in a deeper, more real way. They want to feel their own sexual desire, to stop feeling like they have to perform in bed, and to have a genuinely pleasurable experience of sex.

But maybe that's not you. Maybe you've already got the Grade A super-octane sex life of your dreams. No worries, if so. I'm not in the business of convincing anybody to practice Slow Sex; the choice is truly yours. That said, if your partner dragged you here, that alone may be a sign worth paying attention to! Either way, if you do decide to give it a whirl, try to be open to what happens. You might be surprised. OM is not about going from a "bad" sex life to a "good" one. It's about going from wherever you are to someplace even better. OM can become just one more delightful item on the sexual menu, or it can become a gateway to an even deeper possibility of sexual fulfillment. Either way, I would encourage you to keep an open mind. You never know what you might discover.

Yeah, no. This definitely isn't for me. It happens all the time—people will literally research OneTaste for months, call and have long talks with our coaches, decide they want to learn how to OM, fly across the country, lie down for their first session, and before the stroking even begins decide, "Nope, this isn't for me." The same thing happened to me when I started to OM. I took a few classes and was in and out of the practice for about nine months. Then, one day, without warning, I ran. I ran as far away as I could, burning everything in my wake. I mean, it was *bad*.

It took about six months for me to have my "a-ha" moment about OM. *Oh. It's not the practice I have a problem with. It's that OM is going to change me in ways I'm not sure I'm ready to change.*

I guess I don't have to tell you the end of that story, except to say that my friends and teachers were very kind when I came crawling back on hands and knees, asking for forgiveness and more instruction.

I could tell you this story a hundred times. Yoga, meditation—you name it, I've come up with a reason to avoid it. Just about everything that has changed my life for the better came to me tied up in a big red ribbon of aversion. What I've discovered over the years is that I'm not alone; we humans seem to have a tendency to loathe the very things that have the power to transform us. It's perfectly natural, and even expected.

So you don't want to do the practice—then don't. It's really up to you. But as the saying goes, the opposite of love is not hate; it's indifference. If your response to the idea of OMing is without any sort of charge whatsoever—a true "I could take it or leave it" response—then there might not be anything here for you. If, however, your response is, "No way am I doing something as stupid/ridiculous/outrageous as *that*," then I'd just suggest you take a little peek under the hood and see what's driving your resistance. If I am any example, you might be surprised by what you find.

I hate to be rude, but if it's not about climaxing, then what's the point? It's true: by comparison to our experience of "regular sex," the idea of OM seems strangely anticlimactic. We're not trying to get our rocks off, and we're not trying to wow our partner with our mad sexual talent. We're not doing it as quid pro quo—that is, "I'll have sex with you if you promise to fix the patio door"—and there is no guarantee that you're going to get anything out of the process other than a few moments of (hopefully) enjoyable sensation. Is that all it's about?

It's not. It's about that, but so much more. Because what those few moments of (hopefully) enjoyable sensation show us is a world of possibility beyond. What would it mean to be as in tune with every sensation in our lives as we are with the point of contact between the finger and the clit during an OM? What would it look like if we were able to *feel* our world rather than merely think about it? If we were to be intimate with our partner in a way that put us inside of their experience, instead of trying to understand it from the outside? If our desires were our guiding light, our beacon, our compass? All this begins with connection— connection that we can taste, often for the first time, when we slow down long enough to OM. If we experience that much sensation from just one stroke, what could happen if we put even more effort into connecting with our partners, our friends, and our lives?

This is the question I leave my students with at the end of the Slow Sex workshop. That, and the Ten-Day OM Starter Program in the chapter that follows. It's the best I can do for these sexual artists: sending them into the kitchen with a few ingredients—and then crossing my fingers that I've taught them well enough that the recipe will reveal itself.

Chapter Five

The Ten-Day
OM Starter Program

I designed the Ten-Day OM Starter Program with two hopes in mind. First, I wanted to set specific, easy-to-reach goals that would help new students begin and maintain an OMing practice on their own at home. While students who live near our centers in San Francisco and New York have access to face-to-face coaching and a number of different OMing courses, many of our students are learning from afar. I've found that a day-by-day program is the best way to encourage regular practice, eventually leading them to make OM a part of their everyday lives. The same can happen for you.

The second reason I designed this program is to help you explore some of the more nuanced aspects of OMing—things like communication, stroke direction, pressure, and speed—in an experiential way. I can talk all day about how much pressure a stroker may or may not want to use, but the best teaching is to actually start stroking and asking for feedback.

So you can think of this program as a ten-day prescription for OMing. I can't promise it will cure all your ills, but at the very least I can assure you that if you follow it faithfully, you'll know how to OM on the other end. At most, you'll have found the key to sustainable happiness in your relationship and beyond. Not a bad risk/reward ratio, is it?

For your part, the commitment is just forty-five minutes a day. When I say *just* forty-five minutes in class, the students start to look a bit grumpy and discouraged. Do I not have children? Have I not heard of the sixty-hour workweek? Do I not realize how much time it takes to make breakfast, pack lunches, go to work, make dinner, watch *Mad Men*, squeegee the shower door, floss teeth, apply lip balm? Can I please help them see how they're supposed to be able to cram forty-five minutes of OM practice into their already crazy routine, because they're having a hard time on their own. I used to get a little grumpy and discouraged myself at their resistance. Here I was, offering them the opportunity to try OM, a practice that had genuinely transformed my own life and my relationship to my sexuality, and they were trading it for *Mad Men*?!

Then I started Netflixing *Mad Men*, and I understood the dilemma.

I also remembered something one of my first OM teachers told me. At the time, I myself had been avoiding my own OMing practice. That teacher told me that we *human beings have a universal tendency to loathe what is in our best interest*. In other words, the things that are most potentially transformative, that can heal us in the ways we most desperately desire to be healed; these are the things we most often have to wrestle ourselves to the ground over. Lifestyle changes like yoga, meditating, eating right, and setting aside time to pursue our creative purpose. The

things that seem so hard to squeeze into our busy sched-
ules, even though we know we'll feel *so much better* if
we do.

Things like—I'll go ahead and volunteer—OMing.

So when I suggest that they simply look at how they're
spending their time now—that I'm sure they'll be able to
find the forty-five minutes in there, somewhere—they start
to see me as a drill sergeant at Sexual Bootcamp. What I've
discovered, however, is that there are worse things than
taking my students firmly in hand and forcing them to do
something that deep down they actually really want to do:
make time for sex; return to their bodies and this moment;
dive into a sea of sensation; offer and receive pleasure.
Breathe. Feel. Connect.

Not that getting my students to agree to try the program
means my work is done; I also want them to *complete* the
program. And I speak from personal experience when
I say we all know what it's like to enthusiastically jump
into a new diet, exercise regime, or creative endeavor—
and then watch the commitment fade on day two, when
parent-teacher conferences and flu bugs and last-minute
meetings start to creep back into the mix. The only thing I
can do is remind the students that the OM Starter Program
is only a ten-day commitment, with nothing more required
or expected. Though my secret hope is that they'll come
out on the other side with a burning desire to set up a
daily OM practice, that part is really up to them. It's not
a requirement or even an expectation. All I ask is ten little
days, forty-five minutes a day. Perhaps you can borrow that
time from something that you know is not furthering any
sort of goal in your life. May I suggest TV watching? Imagine me putting my hands on your shoulders and firmly

ou down as I say the following sentence: *Anything*
watching on TV can be DVR'd or downloaded on
r Hulu. You don't have to watch it today.
ays. Ten days is all I'm asking.
od? Good. Let's get down to business.

The Ten-Day OM Starter Program

Each day during the Starter Program I'm prescribing:

- two 15-minute sessions of OMing, plus sharing frames
  with your partner after each
- ten minutes of journaling

What time of day you do the OMing sessions is your
choice. In an ideal world, I would suggest bookending
your day—a session as soon as you and your partner are
up in the morning, and another one before you go to bed
at night. This is, of course, practical only for those couples
who are currently co-habitating. If you are planning to
practice with your boyfriend who lives twenty-four minutes away except in morning rush hour when it's thirty-
six minutes, I'm going to take a flyer and say you might
want to consider doing both sessions back to back. There
is nothing wrong with two back-to-back sessions of OM,
by the way. In fact, it's one of my favorite ways to practice
because it gives you the chance to see how different one
session can be from the next. Sometimes the first session
will be spectacular—over-the-top-orgasmic like nothing
you've ever felt before. Your stroker is a genius! A wizard
of the forefinger! The connection was so rich and nourish-

ing you wonder why the two of you even ever have regular sex anymore, since the true experience you've been looking for all your life is clearly only to be found here, in Slow Sex. Life can't get much better than this.

And then comes session two. Which is sort of...so-so.

As you'll soon discover during the ten-day program, there's a lot of room for "meh" in OM practice. Luckily, there's a lot of room for "spectacular," too. The key is not to judge yourself or your partner too harshly for the so-so session or lavish too much praise for the awesome one. We're just riding the waves here.

"The best OM we've ever had came right after one of the most boring OMs we've ever had. In the first session it felt like unremarkable sex. It felt fine, but nothing special. I thought, 'Well, some days it's just like that.' But as soon as we got up, he suggested we try again. I said okay, and from the minute he put his finger down it was like my body filled up with sparkly light. I think of that feeling as the 'sunshine orgasm.' It was incredibly intense and pleasurable for both of us. We kept saying, 'Whoa! This is crazy!' At one point we both just started laughing out loud because it was just too weird that we could have two such different OMs right in a row." —Ellie, 38

The second step—journaling—gives us the chance to record the experiences we've just had, be they spectacular or *meh*, so we don't forget them. There is no need to overdo it here; I suggest taking a minimalistic approach to the journaling component, at least at first. There's a way that we can freak ourselves out a little bit if we overachieve on the first day—when we feel so inspired we decide to do four sessions of OM instead of two and write eighteen pages of commentary afterward. There's kind of no place to go after that, my friends. More New Year's resolutions die each year from such early flameout. Be the tortoise, not the hare. Be the tortoise.

In other words, set your bar low and raise it from there if you feel inspired to do so. At the beginning, keep it to

- two 15-minute OM sessions
- a few minutes to share frames with your partner
- ten minutes of journaling

Focusing

Each day of the Ten-Day OM Starter Program includes one basic OM session—the technique as it was laid out in the previous chapter—and one "focus" OM designed to help you nail (so to speak) a particular aspect of OMing. Though on one level OM is simply stroking, on another level there are many nuances within each stroke—things like direction, pressure, speed, communication, and more. By isolating just one of these different facets of OM and focusing on it for a fifteen-minute session, we should be able to see how it affects the overall practice. Some practitioners end up loving these focused OMs—the "One-Stroke" OM becomes a favorite for many women, for example—so feel free to incorporate them in your ongoing practice. (The ongoing practice I'm really not pressuring you to commit to at this time but which I secretly hope you'll decide to take up once you see how much happier and more satisfied you and your partner become after you graduate from OMing bootcamp.) (Or not.)

Journaling

I'm not sure why, but some people who take to the OM practice get performance anxiety when it comes to journaling. The inner editor comes and sits on their lap, commenting on the positive or negative nature of every single word that goes onto the page. The way to get around this nefarious voice of evil doom is to never lift the pen off the page for the entire ten minutes you will be writing. (If you're all twenty-first century and prefer to use a computer, this means trying not to pause while your fingers fly across the keyboard. Leave the spell-check for later. For now, just write.) Make your primary goal to write down as many words as possible before the end of the ten minute-session. And remember: nobody else will be reading this journal. It is simply a way for you to further integrate the experiences you've had during your OMs, and then—this is the fun part—to watch your own progress over the course of the ten-day program (and/or beyond).

If you find yourself stuck, unable to think of anything at all to write, use your ten minutes of writing to answer these three questions:

1. What frames did you share with your partner from today's practice?
2. How was the first OM session today different from the second? Compare and contrast, as your ninth-grade English teacher might say.
3. What sensations can you feel in your body right now?

Day One of the OM Starter Program:
Basic OM Practice

focus is simply to practice the basic OMing technique mes second nature. Use the basic OM outlined in us chapter (refer to the OM checklist on pages 97–99 inder) for two fifteen-minute sessions. Be sure to ame with your partner after each session.

Day One Practice

Session 1: Basic OM practice, 15 minutes + sharing frames
Session 2: Basic OM practice, 15 minutes + sharing frames
Journaling: Set a timer for ten minutes, and journal about today's OM sessions. What did it feel like to have two sessions in one day? Did you feel more confident during the second session, or less? How were they different from one another? What did you feel during the OMs? Any other thoughts today, your first day of the Starter Program?

Day Two: Location, Location, Location
(aka Clitoral Mapping)

Now that you and your partner are comfortable with basic OMing, we're ready to start exploring. Day two's focus is all about location—or what is more technically referred to as "Clitoral Mapping." The idea is for both partners to get to know her clit—up, down, and sideways. How it works, where her best "spot" is, and the different sensations that arise depending on where she is stroked. The idea is that once both of you know how she's wired, so to speak, you can use the location of the stroke to help draw out the most possible sensation during your OMing.

The process of Clitoral Mapping is simple. Over the course of the fifteen-minute session, the stroker will stroke at different points around his partner's clit. Each time he strokes a different region, he will tell her where he's stroking and ask her what sensations she feels. Depending on how sensitive and precise the stroker chooses to be, there would be an infinite number of different locations where he might stroke. So to simplify things for the purpose of today's focus, imagine that her clit is the face of a clock, with "twelve o'clock" signifying the top of the clit (from her perspective) and "six o'clock" signifying the bottom. Try to stroke each of the "hours" on the clock at some point during the OM. Feel free to try them in order or, if you're feeling intrepid, jump from one side of the clock to the other. The idea, again, is to stroke a little bit, tell her where you're stroking, and then ask her what sensations it produces in her. "I'm stroking at about seven o'clock. What do you feel when I stroke here?" Together, the two of you will be exploring heretofore uncharted territory—the territory of her clit, her sensations, and her orgasm.

Day Two Practice

Session 1: Basic OM practice, 15 minutes + sharing frames
Session 2: Clitoral Mapping, 15 minutes + sharing frames
Journaling: Set a timer and write for ten minutes about the Clitoral Mapping session. What about it surprised or spoke to you? What were your favorite stroking

locations? Your least favorite? Why? How was the Clitoral Mapping OM different from the "basic" OM you did
today? How are you feeling about the Starter Program in
general, from the vantage point of day two?

"There is a spot on my partner's clit that we jokingly
call the 'love spot.' When I stroke her there, we're both
flooded with these intense feelings of love. We figured it
out through Clitoral Mapping. If we'd simply experienced
an occasional welling up of those feelings in our OMs, we
may have wondered (or mistaken) the meaning. Now we
know, "Oh, it's just the 'love spot.'"   —Joe, 44

Day Three: Speaking Sensations

During yesterday's Clitoral Mapping exercise, the receiving
partner got some practice speaking her sensations. Today,
the stroker gets to join in. In the Speaking Sensations OM,
you will take turns naming the sensations you feel in your
body as the session unfolds. You should be talking contin-
uously throughout the OM, alternating between the stroker
and the receiver. This kind of communication keeps us
present, connected to the sensation, and calibrated to one
another's body. It also helps flex the muscles of communication that are so important in OM—and in intimacy in
general.

Begin with the stroker. Name a sensation you're feeling
in your body. Do your insides feel like maple syrup, velvet, an electric current? Is it more like the color red or the

color blue? Is it steely or watery? Sharp like the blade of a knife or soft and diffuse, like silk? Is it misty like fog or crisp, like bright sunlight? Once you've named your sensation, ask your partner what she's feeling. She may answer right away or she may feel free to pause and really make contact with her sensations before speaking. There is no rush, but stay in verbal contact near-continuously throughout the OM.

At first, my students find the idea of the stroker naming his sensations to be perplexing. How could he be feeling anything orgasm-relevant, given that he's not the one having the orgasm? All I can say is that this is your assignment and I'm sticking to it. Both partners will speak what they are feeling throughout the practice. The experience will serve you later.

Don't be surprised if you—and I'm talking to you strokers especially—have a hard time nailing down a particular sensation. As discussed in chapter 2, we don't have much practice at feeling our bodies deeply enough to be able to locate, investigate, and then name a sensation. But practice makes perfect, and you have many chances to practice right here in this very OM. When in doubt, start with the stroke. What are you feeling in your finger as you stroke? Does your finger feel warm or cool? Dense or feather-light? Does it seem to be rising or falling? Then, pull back the lens until you are able to ask the same questions of your body as a whole. What is happening in your back, your neck, your heart? Do you feel a tingling in your feet, a tightness in your chest, a reservoir of warm liquid pooling in your lower back? Whatever you're feeling say it—and then ask your partner what she is feeling.

Day Three Practice

Session 1: Basic OM practice, 15 minutes + sharing frames

Session 2: Speaking Sensations OM, 15 minutes + sharing frames

Journaling: Set a timer for ten minutes and write about today's sessions. How did speaking your sensations change your experience? Did you find it easy or hard? Comfortable or uncomfortable? Natural or forced? Did you like hearing so many of your partner's sensations? Why or why not? Did you feel more or less connected to your partner when you were speaking sensations than during the "basic" OM session? How would your "regular" sex life change if you were to bring more communication into the mix?

Day Four: Up, Up, Up
(aka the All-Upstroke OM)

One of the most fun and powerful aspects of stroking we can work with is the direction of the stroke, as you'll see through today's focus. The directions we work with in OM are up and down (sorry, no side-to-side here) and direction is determined both by the pressure of the stroke and by the intention of the stroker. If you are meaning to stroke primarily upward, you will use slightly more pressure on the upstroke than on the downstroke. You'll find that if you set your intention to stroke upward, the pressure adjustment will happen naturally: your upstrokes will naturally get more pronounced, and your downstrokes will fade to the background. Decide you want to use downstrokes, and the opposite will take place. When I talk about "pressure," note that I'm not talking about digging deep. Think subtle. You'd be surprised how much difference even a slight change of pressure can make.

Direction has an almost magical effect on the way we feel in our bodies when we're being stroked. As mentioned previously, today's focus will show you just how fun it can be to play with direction. I said this because upstrokes tend to generate sensations of buoyancy and uplift in the body. (Those are fancy words for "fun.") Upstrokes have the ability to make us feel like we, ourselves, are going up, up, up. It's as if each stroke fills us up with a little more helium, carrying us higher into the clouds, the stratosphere, and even right to the moon. Sounds pretty great, no? Might make you wonder why we don't make every OM an "All-Upstroke OM." Our first inkling might be to go straight up as fast and high as possible, every time. But what you may discover through today's focus is that although a quick ascent can be thrilling, the descent comes just as quickly. Like any quick, impromptu fuck, stroking quickly to the heights offers intense sensation—followed by a long slide back down. It has its place, for sure. But over the long haul there is more energy, enjoyment, and nourishment available if we go more slowly. So the point of test-driving the All-Upstroke OM today is both to experience the power of direction firsthand, and also to start the process of discovery that can lead to what I call the "art of continuous ascent." Because there is a sweet spot to be found, a pace at which we can keep stroking upward for fifteen minutes or an hour or even a lifetime without ever hitting the peak. This is what we call "stroking for sustainable up." Try to catch the place where the thrill sensation is starting to crest and wane, and change the stroke momentarily to allow breathing room before continuing upward. Over time, we learn to anticipate that the peak is coming and vary the stroke so we can keep going up.

But for today, don't worry about making it sustainable; just experience it together with your partner. Strokers, practice stroking upward throughout the session. Begin slowly and lightly, adjusting your pressure to continue the energy running upward throughout the session. Remember: a little intention goes a long way. You're keeping your finger on her clit for both strokes, just giving a little bit more emphasis to the upstroke than the down. Listen to your partner; if she is feeling any discomfort with the continuous up, feel free to shift the stroke down for a few moments. The point here is not to stroke upward unfailingly and without respite, especially not if your partner is writhing with overstimulation. Receivers, this is a great place to put the skill you honed yesterday—the skill of speaking your sensations—to work. Both of you will learn more if you talk to each other about what you're feeling as you stroke yourselves right up to the sexual peaks and beyond.

Day Four Practice

Session 1: Basic OM practice, 15 minutes + sharing frames
Session 2: All-Upstroke OM, 15 minutes + sharing frames
Journaling: Write for ten minutes about the All-Upstroke OM. How did it make you feel? Would you want to do an All-Upstroke OM again? Why or why not? Write down the frames you and your partner shared. You'll thank me later: further down the line, when you're wise and savvy OMers, you'll wish you could recapture your first experience of the mighty upstroke.

Day Five: Going Down
(aka the All-Downstroke OM)

Today's focus is going to give you a sense of what it feels like to stroke or be stroked *downward* throughout the session. Most students report that whereas upstrokes bring a sense of headiness, euphoria, and buoyancy, downstrokes have a rich, earthy, grounded quality to them. In a world where we seem always to be chasing the highs and avoiding the lows, there is something especially rocking (that's a technical term) about a practice where success requires *descent* instead of *ascent*. Then there's the fact that an All-Down OM can be a wonderfully sensational, nourishing, delicious experience in and of itself. We so rarely just let ourselves sink down into the sexy earthiness of our bodies that a fifteen-minute mud bath of sorts is sometimes just what the doctor ordered.

Just as with the up OM, begin slowly. You may want to massage her legs before stroking, kneading her thighs and calves very deliberately to help her sink into the feeling sense in her body. When you begin stroking, use a more attentive touch than usual. Not too hard, but not too soft, either. Stroke her downward with broad, meaty strokes, perhaps using the whole pad of your finger instead of the tip. Ask her how she's feeling, and adjust the stroke based on the feedback she gives you. Allow yourself to really go where the stroke is asking you to go. We can sometimes resist plumbing the depths for fear of what might be lurking. Notice and then let go of any resistance you might be feeling. Let the waves of the down wash over you both. There's little in this world more satisfying than the weighty heaviness of down. It's like being insanely hungry and having a huge juicy steak set in front of you. Don't forget to taste every delicious bite.

Day Five Practice

Session 1: Basic OM practice, 15 minutes + sharing frames
Session 2: All-Downstroke OM, 15 minutes + sharing frames
Journaling: Set your timer and write for ten minutes about your experience of the All-Downstroke OM. Did you find it satisfying, neutral, awful? How did it compare to yesterday's All-Upstroke version? If you had to describe the sensation of "down," what adjectives would you use? Again, write down the frames you and your partner shared for this OM—you'll be informed—and likely amused—by them at a later date.

Day Six: Playing with Pressure

Now that your explorations have taken you both up and down, the next step is to investigate the power of pressure. Pressure, like direction, can have a major impact on the sensations that both partners feel during an OM. Used consciously, it's one of the best tools a stroker has to keep sensation increasing over the course of the session.

At the risk of a pun, pressure can be a sensitive issue. Too much pressure, coupled with too much speed, can result in the numbness that is one of the top complaints I hear from female students about their "regular" sex lives. The harder/faster paradigm works wonders for the male apparatus, but it can be deadening to our lacy lady parts. As soon as I say this in class, however, a lot of well-manicured hands go up. These women, for their part, really *enjoy* hard and fast during sex. And I'm sure they do; I know I did. But then I started OMing regularly, and suddenly a whole new world of nuance was mine for the enjoyment. I had become accustomed to a clit that was numbed out or somewhat raw after sex—I didn't even see anything wrong with it, because I had always believed that was what to expect with sex. So I was surprised to discover that my clit was more nuanced, more sensitive, and more capable of picking up subtle sensation *after* OMing than before. And whereas at first I craved more pressure, as time went on I developed an exquisite ability to get off on even the lightest stroke.

In other words, pressure is rich territory for your exploration. Applied in the right places, heavier pressure can offer many of the same qualities as downstrokes: earthiness, pleasant heaviness, and rich satisfaction. Lighter strokes, on the other hand, can add featherweight buoyancy. Today, your assignment is simply to play with both. Start off heavier, until it feels like the OM has ignited. Then switch to lighter strokes, and see how the quality of sensation changes. Be sure to exercise your communication muscle. Strokers, prepare your partner before you up the pressure or switch to a lighter stroke. This not only reminds her to pay attention (minds are built to wander, after all), but it also keeps her from getting surprised by a remarkably strong stroke. Both partners should also now be adept at naming sensations they're feeling during the practice. Though we haven't technically arrived at the lesson about making offers and requests (coming up on day eight), feel free to make use of the Yes/And communication skills you learned in chapter 3. If you want him to stroke with more pressure, say so. If you want to know if you can stroke her even more lightly, don't hesitate to ask.

Day Six Practice

Session 1: Basic OM practice, 15 minutes + sharing frames

Session 2: Playing with Pressure OM, 15 minutes + sharing frames

Journaling: Set your timer for ten minutes and write about your experience playing with pressure during today's OM. How much of a difference could you sense between the heavier strokes and the lighter ones? Did you have a preference for one over the other? If you had that OM to do over again, what might you do differently? How has pressure played into your "regular" sex life, and did you get any insight from today's focus about how you might want to use it differently?

Day Seven: Setting the Pace (aka the Speed-Stroke OM)

Just like pressure, speed is one of the most misunderstood qualities in sex. From the way sex is portrayed in the media, you'd think faster was always better. But that's only because faster makes for more entertaining visuals. Anyone who's tried the slow route knows that the best sex of all is the kind where you don't want to move—not even an inch. Where the sensation is so incredible and you're so connected to your partner that you just want to savor whatever it is you're feeling right now, in whatever position you're in. *That's* the kind of sex we're all looking for, the kind where we can feel every sensation as it rises and falls, like a piece of chocolate melting on the tongue.

Today you're going to explore the territory of speed. Strokers, I want you to use the sensations in your own body as much as your partner's feedback to determine when to apply a faster stroke and when to go more slowly. A faster stroke quickens the heart. Too fast feels like trying to catch a train that left without you. Slowing the stroke gives a temporary exhale, a much needed breather. But go too slow and you'll feel like nothing's shaking—like you're standing around waiting for something to happen. Play around with all of these different feelings, speeding up here and slowing down there. Tell your partner what to expect as you change pace, and tell her about the sensations the shifting of speed brings up in your body. Then ask her what she's feeling, and really listen. Men tend to be very surprised by how much sensation they can create even at a very slow pace. Learn how to put speed to use, and you'll soon be making the most of every single stroke.

Day Seven Practice

Session 1: Basic OM practice, 15 minutes + sharing frames
Session 2: Speed-Stroke OM, 15 minutes + sharing frames
Journaling: Write for ten minutes about your two OM sessions. How did the quality of the Speed-Stroke OM differ from the basic practice? What about the difference between the faster stroking and the slower stroking? Were you surprised by your experience of speed? In what ways? Did you have a preference for slower or faster stroking? What was it like to communicate with your partner around speed?

Day Eight: Making Offers and Requests

Today you'll hone the communication skills you've already been working with by practicing making offers (if you're the stroker) and requests (if you're the receiver). Start with one session of basic OM practice, paying special attention to your own desire. Are there moments when your stroker shifts the stroke in a way that diminishes sensation instead of increasing it? If so, were you willing to make the request that he go back to the more sensational stroke? Most receivers start off hesitant to really communicate their requests to their stroker. As women, we are conditioned to a "take what you can get" relationship with sex. We might be emboldened enough to ask for certain larger things— oral sex, or a particular position that we like—but when it comes to the subtleties of motion, pressure, and speed, we tend to keep to ourselves for fear of insulting the admittedly fragile egos of our beloved men. For their part, said men are reluctant to ask for direction from us for fear of looking like they don't already know—just know, without having to ask—exactly what they're doing. So we end up with the men powering through and the women acting as if. Today, that dynamic gets put to rest.

Guys, your secret is out: she *knows* you don't always know what you're doing. Ladies, if there's one thing that surprised me when I first got into the business of being a sex mentor it was the discovery of just how much men desire our feedback, because it helps them please us. So both of you—start talking.

Today you will take turns making offers and requests throughout the OM. Strokers, use the construction we cov-

ered in chapter 3—"Would you like me to stroke faster/
slower/softer/firmer?" This way, she's either affirming that
you're already doing a great job or she's giving you specific
feedback you can put to use immediately. Receivers, don't
forget to tell him something that feels great—the pressure
he's putting on your leg, his hand underneath your ass, the
location of the stroke—before you make your request. Then,
use the same "Would you..." construction. You're not asking
him if he *can* stroke a little more softly—of course he can,
he's perfectly capable of it—you're asking him if he'd be *willing* to. It may seem like a small difference here on the page,
but it feels completely different in practice. Alternate making
requests and offers, aiming for three to five communications
per partner over the course of the fifteen-minute session.

Note that you can never practice this focus enough.
Making offers (for him) and requests (for her) is a reversal of the gender messages we've been given by society.
Women are conditioned not to ask for too much; men are
conditioned that it's a sign of weakness to stop and ask for
directions. As is the way with Slow Sex, we're in the business of breaking down conditioning and rebuilding our sex
from the foundations. So I encourage you to use this focus
not just today, but as often as you need to until asking and
offering become second nature to both of you.

Day Eight Practice

Session 1: Basic OM practice paying close attention to
any requests and offers you aren't making, 15 minutes +
sharing frames

> **Session 2:** Offers and Requests OM, 15 minutes + sharing frames
>
> **Journaling:** Write for ten minutes about your two OM sessions today. On a scale of 1 to 10, how comfortable do you feel making offers/requests? Did you feel like your partner held up their end of the deal, shifting per your request or giving you the feedback you were asking for? Do you find this kind of communication helpful? Comfortable? Why or why not?

Day Nine: The One-Stroke OM

As I mentioned earlier in the chapter, today's focus—the One-Stroke OM—often becomes a favorite among the women. Its allure has to do with the intense, luscious sensation it produces, yes. But it's also a lot of fun to see just how *surprised* guys are when they realize how very, very slow she actually likes it. The One-Stroke OM is just that: one fifteen-minute stroke from the bottom of her clit to the top and back down again. Strokers, it's up to you to pace yourselves so the stroke lasts the full fifteen minutes. As for pressure, you can vary it however you choose, lighter at some points, firmer at others. The point (outside of sheer enjoyment) is to show, in an admittedly exaggerated way, just how little motion it takes to get a woman off. Compare this single stroke to what markets itself as "great sex" in the media and watch your beliefs about sex start to quiver and quake like—well, like your woman while you're giving her this sensational stroke.

Day Nine Practice

Session 1: Basic OM practice, 15 minutes + sharing frames

Session 2: One-Stroke OM, 15 minutes + sharing frames

Journaling: Write for ten minutes about the One-Stroke OM. What was it like to give or receive such a long, slow stroke? How was it different from the basic OM session? Did it match the expectations you had going in? Would you like to try it again? Why or why not? How might this exercise inform the way you have "regular" sex?

Day Ten: Putting It All Together

So here we are—day ten. If you've made it this far, there's little more I can say. You know how to OM, and you've gotten a taste of all sorts of different strokes. So go ahead, you crazy kids: use the skills you've been practicing the past nine days and have two back-to-back OMs. Try to notice all the different elements you've been playing with during the starter program, from location and sharing sensations to pressure and speed. And don't forget to make offers and requests along the way. Most of all, stay with the stroke and enjoy it!

Day Ten Practice

Session 1: Basic OM practice, 15 minutes + sharing frames

Session 2: Basic OM practice, 15 minutes + sharing frames

Journaling: Go back and re-read your journal entry from day one. How was today's practice different from the first day of the Starter Program? Did the techniques and nuances you practiced these past nine days change your experience of OM? If so, how? Do you expect to continue a daily OM practice now that the Starter Program is complete? Why or why not?

The Secrets of Successful OMers

I promised not to give you the hard sell on continuing your OM practice beyond the starter program, and I intend to keep that promise. The good news is that I really don't have to do very much: most of the couples who make it through the Ten-Day Starter Program do have a desire to continue their OMing practice indefinitely. Whether they actually succeed at getting their practice off the ground is another question. Life has a way of upending even the best-laid plans. But every year, more and more couples are making a daily OMing practice work in their lives. Here are some of the secrets they've shared with me—and I've discovered in my own life:

- **Set a regular time and date to practice.** The number one most important secret to a successful OMing practice is to set up your OM as a recurring appointment. (Hint: you may not want to use your shared office calendar.) Scheduling every single OM can end up feeling like jumping through a whole lot of hoops—after a certain period of time you're bound to get tired and go sit on the sidelines. So make a date and stick to it. Some couples OM every morning before they get out of bed; others do it in the evenings, a couple of times a week. The key is to set the time aside and treat it as inviolable. OM no matter what is going on—whether you just got into a fight or your kid is sick or you'd both rather have "regular" sex that night, commit to OMing and watching what transpires.

- **Keep having "regular" sex—as much as you please.** I meant it when I said that OM is not a replacement for regular sex. One of the top fears I hear from the male halves of OMing couples is that if they start to OM regularly, their women won't want to have sex anymore. While my experience is that the opposite is true, I will still underscore it here: OMing does not replace sex, it improves it. I'll go into the details about just how it can improve your regular sex life in an upcoming chapter. But for now, while you're scheduling your OMs, why not drop a couple of sex dates in there as well?

- **Find a Slow Sex coach.** I remember when I first started trying to meditate at home by myself—it was a disaster. That is, until I found a meditation instructor whom I could call with questions anytime I had them. Slow Sex is the same way: an ounce of support from someone who understands can go a very long way. Couples who come to our courses are assigned Slow Sex coaches, and you can have one, too. We have a team of coaches ready and willing to help you and your partner over the phone or in person. For details on how to find a coach of your very own, visit our website at www.onetaste.us.

Chapter Six

What Men Should Know About Women

Some of the rewards of practicing Orgasmic Meditation can be felt immediately. There's orgasm, of course. There's connection and communication with our partner, a deeper intimacy, a mutual appreciation. There's often an increased appetite for sex, as well as a greater capacity to feel—to feel ourselves, and others, too.

Then there are the rewards that are on a slight delay, the ones we may not even know to look for until we see them unexpectedly blooming all around us. One of the most gratifying—and practical—of these rewards is that it becomes harder and harder to keep our desires to ourselves. Clearly, we all have the desire to see and be seen, to understand and be understood. By the time we get to the end of a Slow Sex workshop the men and the women are voicing this desire to one another. I don't have to plan it; they organically start talking about what they really want from one another, how they are misunderstood, how their needs can be met.

When I first realized this was happening, I decided to make it part of the workshop itself. I separated the men and the women, and gave each group thirty minutes to distill the most important things they ought to know about one another. Then I brought both groups back and had them teach each other—while I took notes. Over the years of doing this exercise, the cream has risen to the top. The best, sweetest, most nourishing desires have emerged over and over until they've become a sort of canon of wisdom about what men and women want. What follows in this chapter and the next are the ten most insightful and surprising discoveries that the men have made about the women, and the ten that the women have made about the men. Some will feel confronting, some controversial. Others will feel like common sense—but the kind that we tend to forget unless reminded. So I hope you will take these suggestions as reminders, conversation starters, and a jumping-off point for your own orgasmic exploration. The collective wisdom gathered here has served me in many ways over the years, and I am honored to be able to share it with you now.

1. **For women, everything is connected.** Her body and her heart and her sex. Her work and her relationships and her journey. Her world looks like a spiderweb, with everything intimately tied to everything else. Your world looks sleek and organized and flawlessly direct; even your sexual organs are elegantly packaged and compartmentalized on the exterior. Hers are inside of her, literally sharing space with her stomach and her guts and her heart. Take note of that difference, and you may understand how to share a bed, and a life, with her. You may suddenly understand why sex can never be merely sex: it's right there in the middle of the full catastrophe. For a woman, there is no such thing as separate. Sex is food is love is spirit. It's why sex makes her cry. It's why, when something

goes wrong in some other very different area of her life, it can feel like something has gone wrong in her sex life, too. She is interwoven and lovely and sometimes messy and often complex. She is like a kaleidoscope, and her body works the same way. Touch her in one place and she'll feel it in ten others. Circumambulate her most sensitive parts, exploring the outer reaches before going in for the treasure. And go slowly, slower than you ever thought imaginable. You can't help but draw out her orgasm, a whisper at a time.

2. **Women want to have sex just as much as men—just not the sex that's on the menu.** Perhaps that's overstating it. She likes the sex on the menu, she's just not hungry for steak every single day. Women crave variety and surprise and spontaneity; we want a seasonal menu, a specialty menu. We want items that arouse and nourish and satisfy every part of us, because every part of us is connected to every other part. We want hot sex and we also want smooth, silky sex; we want climactic sex and we want slow, undulating sex. We want range. We want gradients. We want sex to move from slow to fast, from hard to exquisitely soft. We want to be surprised by nuance and subtlety. We want the chance to go up and then come back down, not just once but over and over. We want to communicate our sensations and hear about yours.

Do not believe us if we say we do not want sex; we want sex more than you guys could possibly fathom. We are, quite literally, starved for the feeling of orgasm in our bodies. But we haven't been given permission to discover the unique sensations of our own orgasm, so we don't know how to order what we desire. In this, we need your help. We need you to help get us turned on, to unfreeze us and get our waters flowing again. Give us the time, space, and permission to taste a bite of every possible sensation and to communicate which ones we like and which ones we could do without. Show us—telling us is not enough—that you are not bored by the kind of sex that warms us from the inside out. OM with us. Touch us slowly. Ban the rule of reciprocity for a night or two, so we don't have the excuse of worrying about your orgasm to keep from dropping down into our own. In exchange, you will gain access to a whole world of turn-on—ours. You will be matched, finally, by a woman who can truly feel what she wants. Who can get off on hard-fast-hot and guide you toward nourishing-hydrating-expanding all in one delicious evening.

3. **Women will short-order their desires**. For many reasons, and with many painful results, women have been conditioned not to eat, even when we are hungry. Hungry for food, hungry for love, and—most devastatingly for you—hungry for sex. We have been taught that good women tame their desires, don't even feel them; that pushing through our hunger is good and giving into it is bad. As a result, your woman will tend to short-order her desires, be they for connection or food or sex. She will order what she thinks she's supposed to want, divided by half. She won't even explore her options because she already knows what she's allowed to order and what she's not. And she'll always leave a few bites on her plate.

In other words, your woman will be running on empty. And running on empty is not what you want your woman to be, unless you like irritability, impatience, hypersensitivity, and for everything to be your fault. Because in the space between what she asks for and what she really wants, resentment will begin to fester. And you, sir, will be the one she blames.

Find out what she is hungry for, and give it to her. Never accept her first answer. Ask again. And again. Make it part of your game plan to prod and push until she releases what she is withholding and her desire comes flying out. At first, her desire might sound like anger. She may need to blow off steam. Don't take it personally, even if she says hurtful things.

Keep asking until you feel her true desire release. You will feel it in your body when she finally lets go. Regardless of how much resistance she has, don't stop asking until you feel it. You are helping her unravel a lifetime of conditioning—old beliefs and habits and rules that are suffocating the bright, lovely, sexy woman within. *That's* the woman you want to be with. So if you have to ask all night, ask all night. You'll know it when she finally speaks her desire because you will be able to feel it, landing with a satisfying *thunk* in your body.

Then give it to her, and you'll be giving her the thing she never thought she could get: not just the desire, but approval for having the desire at all.

"I was surprised to find that other people noticed changes in me after we started OMing. I hadn't told anyone I worked with that we were doing a sex practice, of course. People just saw me change. I heard comments like 'You look great!' 'You're smiling more,' and 'You look more at ease and happier than I've seen you before.' I was amused but of course I didn't dare say what was different. I just noted how this kind of comment kept coming up over and over."

—Donna, 49

4. **Women have as much sexual energy as men, it just freezes more easily.** <u>Sexual energy is life energy</u>; we all have it. Women don't have less of it than men; it's just that ours gets frozen more often. Body image, previous relationships, something her dad said to her when she was eleven—by the time you meet her she may be so iced over that only a trickle of desire is getting through. Without regular access to the warm heat of orgasm, the freeze gets deeper and deeper until she has no more access to her desire at all.

The problem is that when her desire is frozen, everything else starts to feel frozen, too. Her body. Her heart. Her pussy. Everything is connected, remember? So the sexual energy builds and builds, and there is no place for it to go except deeper within.

The pinch is that <u>the solution—sex—looks like the enemy</u>. It looks like a hard workout on cold muscles, a preamble to a sore and tender everything. Sex is so potent, and she is so frozen, she fears it will shatter her on impact. So instead of moving closer to the heater, she huddles farther and farther away, off-gassing the energy in a thousand little ways: picking fights, throwing barbs, casting blame.

Help her thaw out her energy, get it moving again, and she'll start turning on more easily. <u>Listen to her</u> when she is talking so she feels the connection between you. Take a <u>walk with her</u>. <u>Run her a bath</u>. Then <u>OM with her</u>, making sure to <u>ground her</u> with love (and firm pressure) when you are through. OM is like a hot water bottle, getting things all melty and smooth again. Stroke by stroke, you can thaw out all the conditioning that tells her it is unsafe to be a sexual woman, so that her turn-on can flow through unobstructed.

"During and immediately after OMing, I have a sense of energetic movement in my limbs and the core of my body. I feel more relaxed and alert at the same time—more clearheaded." —Petra, 28

5. What she really wants is access to your attention. Men receive lots of messages about what to give a woman to get sex and love in return. Jewelry, fancy dinners, a big house. This is the equivalent of stroking her with lots of speed and pressure. Thrilling and beautiful and appreciated, yes, but it doesn't get to the heart of our desire. When we ask for these things, it's because we've learned to accept them as a proxy for what we *really* want but have never had access to: the animating, enlivening experience of having your full attention placed on us whenever we desire it.

If you want to give her what she really wants, show her that she can have as much of you as she needs. Answer her phone calls, be present when you are having a conversation with her, and make good on your promises. When she realizes you are not a scarce resource, the yowl of her hunger will settle down to a pleasurable purr. Then, the gifts become a choice you make in order to delight her, rather than an obligation you fulfill in order to appease her.

6. Learn to navigate her desire. Women want sex; we are starving for it. We *want* to be turned on. We *want* to follow our desire. We *want* to thaw out and get our energy moving so we can use it for sex and relationship and everything else.

Yet give us a hundred opportunities to have sex, and we'll come up with a hundred good reasons not to.

I'm too tired. The kids aren't asleep yet. I feel fat today. We just ate—aren't we supposed to wait half an hour? I don't have time. I'm on my period. I need my beauty sleep. I'm not in the mood. Didn't I ask you to clean out the basement?

Here's the secret: we have been programmed to keep our sex locked up and hidden. It's not our fault—most of the time we don't even realize we're doing it. Our mothers (and our mother's mother, and *her* mother before that, all the way back to the beginning of time) created us that way, to keep us safe. The script goes like this: *When sex is near, discover an impossibly large obstacle, drag it into the middle of the road, and then blame it for not allowing you to have sex.*

But that's not really what we want. What we really want is to let the sex enter us, liberate us. We *want* the energy and enjoyment and intimacy. We have the desire, we just don't give ourselves permission to feel it.

So you must learn to navigate her desire. This cannot be done via force, bargaining, or guilt. It can be done only by careful, deliberate request. When she says no, ask again. And again. You're not trying to look good here, you're trying to make your woman *happy*. These are two very different results. When she says no, do not turn away in rejection. Instead, look her in the eyes and let her know you see her. You see the desire *and* the obstacles. And then help her clear the latter so the former can flow. Promise to help her do the laundry later in the day (this won't work unless you do it, so *do* it). Make plans to exercise with her in the morning. Use humor and curiosity to penetrate her resistance. Then ask again if now is, in fact, the time to have sex.

You are making it safe for her desire to arise, proving

that you are in her corner. Help her taste her own desire in a way no man has ever taken the time to do before. Then let her desire take over, until she is throwing you down on the bed and you can harvest the rewards of her freedom for your own enjoyment.

7. **Women have no idea how much men love them**. Whatever you place your attention on will reveal its secrets to you, and I've spent a lot of my life attending to men. The secret I've learned after so much time spent with you is this: we women completely, totally, and fatally underestimate your desire to please us.

Forgive us; our reception channel is sometimes full of static. After so long fighting to wrest our so-called power "back" from you, it seems like a cruel joke to discover that you have always loved us. What a surprise. All you can do here is be careful, deliberate, and tenacious about reminding your woman that you love her and you always have. Show her through kindness and humor and a willingness to please her even when she is pushing you away. Take her to dinner, or better yet—make dinner yourself. Rub her feet, go to the movie she wants to see, offer her a cup of tea. Consider yourself a key player in the game of male-female dynamics, and get curious about what your next play should be. And—this is the hardest part—<u>leave behind any resentment</u> you might have accumulated over being accused of a crime you did not commit. Someday, when she finally sees who you've been all this time, she will make it up to you.

8. **Behind every woman's complaint is a desire**. I'm afraid I might lose my card-carrying position as a woman for this

one, but here goes. *Women have been trained to get what we want by playing the role of victim.* We have been frozen in the role of withholding, of being sure we need to fight to get our needs met. Complaining is a prime tactic we use to this end.

But there is a secret, and it is this: behind every woman's complaint is a desire. The complaint is like the perilous moat around the palace of her hunger. Her desire is so tender that she can't reveal it to just anyone. She must know that you will be careful with it, that you really want it, and that you will treat it with dignity. So she's going to make you work for it by presenting it to you as a complaint.

Think of the complaint as the steam rising from a delicious plate of food. The steam is ephemeral, but it still can burn. Pay attention to it, but don't mistake it for something solid in and of itself. It is simply a signal. *There is a luscious, living desire here; come find it.* She will guard it with all her might, so you must disarm her with gentle humor and curiosity. Watch yourself; be vigilant not to turn your humor into barbs. When she complains, ask her gently what desire is behind that. Coax it out of her until she believes you are earnest. Keep the game going, rather than collapsing under the weight of any one complaint. Each complaint is an oyster, with the pearl of desire inside. Go in and find it.

9. Women are not just dishonorable men. My choice of career sent my mother into therapy. She would ask her therapist, why was I trying to kill her? Why was I trying to destroy her life? Why was I turning my back on everything she had ever taught me? Luckily the therapist understood something my mother did not. She explained that it wasn't that I had the same values as my mother and was merely being defiant. It was that I operated by *an entirely different code*. In following my passion, I was being true to my own code.

The same holds for all women. We have not sworn allegiance to your code and then flagrantly disobeyed it. We are loyal to an entirely different code.

We don't mind that you're not like us; we like it when you are earth and we can be sky. We do want you to learn to be flexible, however, like a tree that can stay rooted but still bend in the wind.

If you are confused by something we say, don't take it personally—simply ask us to rephrase. If we do something that goes against your rules and regulations, use it as an opportunity to expand your own range. Resist the temptation to ask the unanswerable question of "Why can't they be like us?" And do not buy into the fantasy of finding a woman who is; she doesn't exist. Consider the strength her tests help foster in you. If you can learn the delicate art of balancing that strength with flexibility, then true mastery will be yours.

10. She doesn't want to win. She doesn't want "her" way, she wants "our" way. She wants to collaborate, to negotiate. They say that in Morocco the street vendors get offended if you accept their first price, because haggling is how you create a bond. It's how you relate, how you create intimacy. Women operate the same way. We want both sides to get a little of what they want, because it is in between "you" and "me" that relationship is created.

We haven't communicated this to you, however, and it does not follow your natural inclination. You are conditioned to be independent. In your world, you decide or she decides. One or the other. So when she gets bent out of shape that you haven't included her, didn't even think to consult her, what you hear is that *she* wants to do it. And so you bow out, thinking that is the way to make her happy. But it does not make her happy. In the move from "ours" to "hers," relationship gets lost. She is left feeling abandoned, and you are left feeling irrelevant.

Don't settle for letting her get her way. Your acquiescence is not valuable to her; <u>what she craves is your participation</u>. She wants to come together with you and make a better decision than either of you would make on your own. There is a very easy way to make her happy here. <u>Always present her with three options</u>. Research three different restaurants you would like to take her to, and then give her a choice. Think of three different times when you might OM together, and let her pick which one. She will feel held by you because you took the time to narrow things down. She will feel respected by you because you let her decide. (Plus you'll always get one of your top three picks, which is more than you could say when you were letting her have her way.)

Chapter Seven

What Women Should Know About Men

It can be tempting to generalize and say that women are demanding and men are at our mercy. But give a thoughtful group of men permission to express the desires that lie hidden in their often-guarded hearts, and what you discover may surprise you. Men are both more complex and easier to understand than most women realize. Here are the top ten things they want us to know—a list that doubles as the top ten ways to keep our beloved men at their absolute best.

1. Men experience acknowledgment through a woman's happiness. People often wonder how I convince men to practice Orgasmic Meditation—as if it would take something just shy of forced inscription to get a man to stroke a woman's genitals for fifteen minutes. Even we women are amazed to discover how willing, even honored, he is to OM with us. We hardly believe it could be this easy. To feed our hunger and to get our needs met have always felt like such a struggle. So at first we are suspicious: *It must be* *because it's sexual. He likes anything sexual. He's still not going to take out the garbage when I ask him to.*

And then they go home, and suddenly he's perfectly willing to take out the garbage.

One of my male students explained it best. "If she's happy, it makes me happier." This is the life-giving secret: *He judges how well he is doing by the happiness of the woman he is with.* The measure of his manhood is how happy *you* are. The happier you are, the happier he will be. When you are turned on, there's nothing he can't do. So OM becomes the best friend he ever had. It is a foolproof way to make his woman orgasmic, and an orgasmic woman is a happy woman.

Lie back and let him draw your orgasm out. There is no need for guilt; this is something he has been waiting for. Allow him to stroke you, and watch him respond in ways you'd never imagined.

> "At first, I would always rather have been having sex or giving him a blow job or doing something that would make *him* feel good, so he would like me more. It was very challenging for me to just lie back and feel. I had this fear that when we were practicing he would realize he didn't love me. But the opposite happened. I have never been able to trust a relationship this much in my life, because now I don't have to guess how he's feeling. When we OM, I can *feel* how he's feeling."   —Sarah, 30

2. If you want him to treat you like an equal, then be his equal. Something I hear often from women is that they withhold sex because sex is the only card they have. They must play it wisely. If they give it away too quickly, or too frequently, they'll have nothing left. He'll have all the cards and what will they do then?

The problem with this strategy is simple. Men do not actually have all the cards. They are only acting as if they do because they think that's what you want. They think you want them to be all-powerful. Guys think that's the only way you'll feel protected, and as far as they can tell, you need protection. If I had a dollar for every time I heard a man say, "I can't tell her that—she couldn't handle it!" I would use that money to buy a billboard over Times Square saying *She is not broken!* The problem is, you *appear* to be broken a lot of the time. If someone has to fill the "alpha" position, it's going to have to be him.

But you are not broken, you protest. You can handle just as much as he can, if not more. (Let *him* try out menstruation and childbirth, and then we'll see who's broken.)

You are right. And yet this is one of the most painful things I have to point out to women: we work very hard to convince others that we just can't do it. We are the queens of the "yes, but…" We are ready at any moment to rattle off a litany of our flaws—all the reasons we are not enough. This works with our women friends; we've long known how to read between the lines. But men take things at face value. If you talk about all the ways you are less than, he starts to believe it.

If, on the other hand, you show him your ability—how whole you can be, how you *can* handle it—then his need to be alpha will subside.

This is key, since one of the greatest hopes of my women students is that their men might learn to show more emotion, to be more intimate, to let them in. Understand that he cannot show you his emotions if you seem to be falling apart all the time. If he is to open to you, you have to first show him that you can handle his emotions. Show him you can hold him.

Once in a workshop a woman was weeping, crying to the point where she could barely speak. She was telling her husband how much it hurt her that he was not more emotional. His response said it all: "How can I be? One of us needs to hold it together."

He is going to do everything he can to maintain equilibrium. If he sees you in a perpetual state of falling apart, he will swing to the opposite pole. If you want him to feel safe letting go, then it's up to you to develop the muscle of steadiness. Your steadiness itself will give him the freedom to show you what is really going on in his heart.

3. Nice is the trump card. I meet so many fantastic women. Women who are smart and sexy, witty and charming. Women with charisma and verve, who can work a ten-hour day and then throw a dinner party for eight without so much as a nap. Women, it seems, who can do anything.

Everything except find and keep their man. They watch the men they desire fall desperately in love with women who aren't as smart, who aren't as sexy, who wouldn't know the first thing about choosing the right wine to go with mole chicken. Women who have accomplished nothing at all with their lives. Why *her*?

When the men are teaching the class and the women ask this question, they are momentarily stunned by the response. It's simple, the guys point out. The woman they go for is the one who is *nice* to him.

The one who loves him. Who he can see appreciates him.

"We would do anything in the world for you," they say, "if we thought it meant you'd be *nice* to us."

All the other credentials pale in comparison. Everything else is icing on the cake, more for your own pleasure than for his. This isn't to say that your accomplishments aren't important. They're what make the experience of being *you* just fun enough that your joy can overflow onto him. But much more important than your credentials is your capacity to feel full enough yourself that you can extend toward him with care. Start with one moment of genuine appreciation, and feel your way from there.

4. Say it to a man every time like the first time. The female ear, like everything else about us, is trained to operate on multiple channels. It's why we can all talk at once and still be understood. It's why we know what she's saying, even when she's *not* saying what she really *wants* to say—because we can hear her on all different levels, even the silent ones.

Men are trained to hear well on one channel at a time. If you come to him with more than one channel broadcasting— saying one thing but meaning another—you will miss your target completely. He will only hear the one you are saying out loud. The same thing is true when it comes to sex. For women, sex is operating on many channels at once. It's about emotion, connection, nourishment, and—sometimes but not always—desire. When you're "doing it," you're "doing it" on multiple levels. Your man, however, is doing it on just one level at a time. Hate to say it, but most of the time he's just "doing it."

The way to bring your two worlds together, whether in

communication or in sex, is to slow down and repeat. Say everything as if you were saying it for the first time. Every stroke a new stroke. Every request a new request. No condescension, no judgment. Just a willingness to start over again in every moment.

5. Fixing is what a man does when he can't figure out how to turn you on. We women have been trained that the only way to get our needs met is to assume the role of victim. To collapse, to break beneath the weight of our unmet desire. Your man wants to help, but all he sees is you, lying there, broken. He does not hear the desire, he hears only the complaint. So he takes the complaint into his little woodshop, pulls out his trusty tools, and commences to fix. To fix the problem. To fix his woman and make her happy again.

But of course, fixing isn't what we want at all. When we're not turned on, what we want is to be *turned on*. Turn-on happens through play. We want to be tempted and teased, not poked and prodded. We want to be held and felt, not told what to do. When he turns to his workbench and begins to tinker away, we accuse him of ineptitude. We feel like he doesn't see us, like he doesn't understand us. In truth, all he's doing is responding to what feels like an emergency in the only way he knows how.

Instead, you can use his fixing nature to inspire your own turn-on. Remember that his tendency to go into handyman mode is his way of saying "I love you." It's all he has. It may be in a foreign language—it may be all consonants and no vowels so it's a bit clunky and awkward—but it is "I love you" nonetheless. Let the love fill you up, turn you on, and then gently redirect him toward your desire.

> "Most men my age don't know how to touch a woman. I don't blame them. They never really learned. So it's been amazing to have my partner touching me in a way that truly feels good for the first time." —Donna, 58

6. His conditioning says for him to be autonomous and independent. For a while at OneTaste, we were teaching a lot of sexuality courses specifically for women. Then one day we got the bright idea to teach a class for men. We called it "What Ten Women Want You to Know," and that's exactly what the guys got: ten real women telling them exactly what they wanted men to know about women.

As you can imagine, there was quite a lot to say.

I moderated the discussion and watched as each of the guys leaned in, silent, not moving a muscle. I've never had such a rapt audience, before or since. I thought we'd struck gold—this was the best, most amazing course we'd ever created. These guys didn't want to miss one word of what we women were telling them.

But then the men left for their lunch break—and didn't come back.

We couldn't figure it out. The guys seemed to *love* the course, giving us their full and complete attention and showing no signs of overload. But then they disappeared before it was over.

I only understood once I stopped thinking of the men as women. Women, who are conditioned to connect in groups, and thus feel comfortable letting their feelings be known to those around them. Who nod when they like what they're hearing and grimace or look away when they don't. From the time we're little girls, we're taught to fly in flocks. So we know how to recognize one another's signs and how to make our feelings known in subtle ways.

I had to start thinking of the men as men, who are trained from a very early age to keep it all in. Who are more comfortable as their own independent entities. These men had no way of letting us know when we were giving them too much information. They didn't think they had a right to tell us they'd had enough, that we were going too far. Instead, they held it all in—and then fled at the first opportunity.

With men, we must go slow and check in frequently. Give lots of breaks, chances for him to blow off some steam. Otherwise long before you notice any signs he may overload and then head for the hills. The lesson is this: one stroke at a time.

And men, if you're wondering what tips we gave out during that class, it all came down to one sweet request: be more you. That's it. Show yourself to us. It's all we've ever wanted.

7. He really is that simple, and it's not the same as dumb. One of my favorite exercises in the workshop is to have the men and women partner up and speak every thought that comes into their minds for two minutes. The women begin, and they have great fun with it. They are dreaming about a new life, or thinking about their girlfriend's wedding, or planning a trip to Mexico, or wondering what is happening with that other couple across the room. When the bell goes off, there is a pained moan. The exercise is over? It went so fast.

Then we have the men start talking.

I said, *then we have the men start talking.* Start talking, men!

Another pained moan, this time because they have nothing to say. Really. What are they supposed to say? When the exercise is over, there is an audible sigh of relief.

The male brain, to the women's amazement, actually seems to be focused on *what he himself is doing right now.* All the delicate nuance that a woman sees happening around her, all the time—it doesn't even make it to his radar. We expect him to be communicating via body language and studied silences. He, on the other hand, has already said everything he needed to say. He couldn't have been more clear. That's why our men become frustrated when we're always asking them to tell us four times what they *really* meant. They *really* meant what they said. Just what they said, and no more. They have been taught to focus. To be straightforward, direct, and honest. They say what they think. Integrity comes before all. So when he doesn't go into detail, do not take it personally. It is not that he doesn't love you, that he can't feel you. It's that he already told you. Go back to his words, and allow their full weight to land within. You may discover you have no more questions at all.

8. When you hit, **it hurts**. Remember the first time you hurt someone you love? You were probably a kid, playing with your little brother or your best friend, and you were horsing around as all kids do. Maybe you were pushing a bit too hard, and you knew on some level that you were crossing a line, but you didn't think any harm would come of it. You had no intention of actually *hurting* him. So when he started to cry—to cry for real, with big juicy tears falling off his eyelashes and down the front of his T-shirt—the pain was like someone was trying to surgically remove your heart without anesthesia.

That's how the women feel in class the day the men tell us how easily, and how often, we hurt them with what we say. The first time I heard a guy say it with such honesty, I think the pang in my chest may have left a scar.

I see this in my coaching as well. For example, a couple takes part in class and the guy won't be saying very much. His partner will say something that could seem innocuous if you weren't listening very carefully, and he'll explode.

"Did you hear that? I just can't take her put-downs anymore!" he'll say. And she'll look at him like he has four heads.

"He *got* that?" she'll be thinking. Most women have no idea that the barbs they send out even land with him. We've learned over the course of time that the only way to get our desires is to try to squeeze them in through the back door. So we start to squeeze a whole lot in through the back door, including—in the case of this couple—a whole lot of our pain. We want it to be acknowledged, but we have never gotten very far with direct communication. So we cloak our true feelings with a joke or a smile or a backhanded compliment.

Until we realize that when we cut him down—even if we do it with a smile on our face—he feels it. In class we do an exercise where throughout the day, the men will raise their hands whenever a woman in class says something that hurts. It's shocking how many hands are in the air, and how often. It's a wake-up call for the women; men actually *feel*! Even though they've been trained not to acknowledge it, to let it run off their backs, to dismiss our commentary as nagging or bitchiness or "that time of the month." In that one exercise, the truth comes out—they feel us, even when we think we're being sneaky. It's a cycle of viciousness: we're being mean because we think he's going to dismiss us if we speak our desires directly; he's dismissing us because we're being *mean*.

The cure is communication. Pure, simple, unobstructed. Start with sex, with OM. Tell him what he's doing right, and ask him if he would do just this one thing a little bit differently. Be neutral. Remember the first rule: what he wants more than anything is for you to be happy, for you to be nice to him. Show him that you're on his side during sex, that you are setting him up to succeed at this life's work, and soon you'll be able to get your desires met in the bedroom and beyond.

9. **Men get confused when women withhold information.** We women are better at strategy than an army general. When we have something important to say, we ruminate on it all day long. We think of twelve different ways we might phrase it in order to get just the response we're looking for. We'll wait and wait for the perfect moment. We'll use all of our energy to hold back. We'll plan out how we're going to use 25 percent fewer words than we really want to—you know, for *impact*. Then we will wait and hold, wait and hold, until we can't keep it inside anymore and we have to let it out.

At which point, without fail, it comes out all wonky and hysterical-sounding. First, because only 75 percent of the information is there. Second, because unexpressed desire has a very short shelf life. When it arises, it's all bright and shiny and perfect. But let it stand out on the counter until "just the right moment," and you can guarantee something that is a little moldy and stinky and soft in the middle.

And then we're surprised when he is upset, or confused, or didn't actually get the message. We did such a good job strategizing! We waited! We used 25 percent fewer words than we wanted to! Maybe we should have sent the third version of the e-mail, instead of the sixth...

It wouldn't have mattered, of course. To decipher whatever message you sent him, in just the way you wanted it to land, would take a world-class psychic. Or a woman. I highly doubt your partner is the former, and if your partner is the latter, you probably have a whole different set of communication issues. (If my own past history is any indication.) Men are trained to relate to the world through *overt* communication, so they are reliably useless at understanding anything we don't actually *say*. It doesn't matter how loud we scream at them from inside our heads. We must communicate in s-i-m-p-l-e, p-l-a-i-n w-o-r-d-s, spoken out loud. The more specific, the better.

This doesn't mean men aren't sensitive beings. As discussed previously, they feel—a lot. Even when they didn't quite understand what you were trying to say, they know if there was something in there that was meant as a dig. It's like when you hold a tuning fork up to a guitar, and the string with the same note will start vibrating. On an unspoken level, he resonates to your frequency. And it hurts.

The secret? He can resonate to your frustration and your confusion and your pain. But he can also resonate to your desire—and respond accordingly. So tell him. Use plain English. Don't hold anything back. And watch him rise to the occasion. It's what a man does best.

10. Approval turns him on. Approval—yours—is all he is looking for. When a man can feel a woman's genuine acceptance of who he is, her pleasure in what he's doing for her, he lights up like the Eiffel Tower. He will immediately try to figure out what he did to deserve it, and he will do that thing again and again in hopes of a similar response. We women think it's so much more complicated than that. But in truth, men love feeling wanted, needed, desired, and appreciated. It's how you get a man to come out of his cave; it's how you show him he "done good." Approval is the fuel that gets the fire inside of him burning brightly.

The hard part is that growing up as a woman, you were probably taught that showing "too much" approval would bring you *unwanted* attention. It would work too well. Or you were taught not to add fuel to his fire of turn-on by showing him how turned on *you* got in his presence. So you learned not to give men a lot of praise, not to let them see the tender part of you that experiences pure, unbridled joy in their presence. You may even have been taught disdain for men who are "too needy," who thrive on praise and compliments. You were not taught the subtle but important difference between false praise and genuine appreciation, a difference he can feel.

So we learned how to keep our own genuine turn-on hidden, all the while manufacturing false turn-on in order to get what we wanted from him. The problem is that in the process, men learned to distrust all of our turn-ons, even the authentic kind. Help him trust you again. Give him the real thing, the stuff you were taught to keep hidden. That's what he wants to feel. When you take the leap and share your turn-on with him, the result is the fire of intimacy you're both secretly craving.

Chapter Eight

Slow Sex, Meet Regular Sex

Let's be honest. When they first find me, most of my students aren't looking for a sexual meditation practice. What they're looking for is better sex. More sex, for starters, but also more depth, more connection, and more orgasmic sensation in the sex they're already having. As it turns out, they get just what they're looking for—but not in the way they expected. Because what I hear over and over from these same students is that once they start to practice, it's OM itself that keeps them practicing. OM is magical in that way; it's impossible to sense, from the outside, what could be so special and amazing about it. But once you experience OM, the nourishment you feel speaks for itself.

The bonus is that this nourishment seeps in and enlivens the rest of your life as well—including and especially your "regular" sex life. It's all connected, after all. Transform your relationship to sexuality in one area, every other area gets touched in the process. So it is that Slow Sex enters the field of "regular" sex: naturally and without any help from you. At the same time, there's no harm in aiding and abetting the process. You can attend to your regular sex life the same way you have learned to attend to sensation during OM. In this case, that means infusing every sexual interaction with the same three Slow Sex ingredients: stripping down, feeling sensation, and asking for what you desire.

It also means learning to savor an experience that we are used to pushing through. When we take climax as our goal—rather than simply feeling each stroke along the way—we tend to crash through sex, picking up speed as we go. It's like we're pushing through a windstorm, striving to reach the finish line. As a result, we miss out on everything that's available to us right now. We don't have time to absorb the sensation we are looking for, and as a result we end up even hungrier than when we started.

> "Before we started OMing, sex was all about the climax. Now both of us have more of an appreciation for the pleasure that comes before. This may mean we mutually decide to end sex before one or both of us climax because we've gotten to a place where we feel really good and we want to carry that energy into the next thing we do. Now sex is less about getting rid of energy than getting it moving, so it becomes fuel for the day."   —Stefan, 37

The antidote to this finishing-line mentality is learning how to hold. Holding means breaking the habit of leaning forward all the time. It means savoring the sensation of the wind against our skin, rather than trying to escape it. Dropping the goal orientation and feeling our orgasm for where it wants to go. Maybe it wants to move toward climax; maybe it doesn't. Either way, we follow its direction.

We let it wind its way, meandering through sensation after sensation, until it's reached its fill. This choice to savor our experience is what puts the "slow" in Slow Sex. We slow down, and all of a sudden we can feel what we weren't able to feel before: we can feel our own desire. Its longing for climax and resolution. Its texture and motion. Everything it is, which *is us*.

Slow Sex vs. Regular Sex

Regular Sex	Slow Sex
Looking good	Feeling good
Guidebooks, rules, and instructions	Native wisdom
Obligation	Desire
Fantasizing	Attention to sensation
Making sex happen	Letting sex happen
Volume	Potency
Increasing sensation through pressure	Increasing sensation through attention
Linear	Meandering
Straining	Easeful or effortless
Relieving the surface itch	Dropping in for deeper fulfillment
Goal of climax	Goal to feel every stroke
Numbness after climax	Nuanced sensation after climax
Myth of insatiability	Experience of filling up
Control	Surrender

A new kind of climax becomes the natural next step—it rolls through you, rather than happening *to* you. With this kind of climax you are present for every stroke as it rises up and through. You're no longer tensed up, contracted, hopeful of getting something. You are relaxed, alert, and connected to your partner as sensation builds, peaks, and goes over. There is an ease to it, like ice gradually melting into water. Gratification becomes available in every moment.

The process of transforming "regular" sex into Slow Sex is, of course, an art rather than a science. It must happen naturally; there is no step-by-step instruction, no technique I can offer. The best I can hope to do is to inspire you, to point you in the right direction. The three exercises that follow are meant to do just that. They illustrate one person's experience—my own—with the "slow" versions of oral sex and intercourse. My hope is that they might ignite within your body that intuition that brought you to Slow Sex in the first place. I invite you to read them, perhaps aloud to your partner. Pay attention to the sensations they create in your body as you go, and take from them any ideas that resonate with you.

Then put this book down. Feel your desire. And let your own unique recipe for Slow Sex reveal itself to you, stroke by stroke.

Slow Sex for Women

Slow Sex, I tell my students, was built for women. Women naturally desire sex that is connected, earthy, sensual, and artistic. We want the permission to be turned on. We want our men to help us reach that goal. The rules for us are only these three:

Go slow. Slower than you could ever imagine. So slow you can feel her, smell her, taste her every cell.

Be unpredictable. Her orgasm responds to the element of surprise. Don't think too hard—just let yourself feel. Follow your own sensation wherever it wants to take you; desire co-arises, so whatever feels best to you will be the path of most sensation for her, too.

Learn to hold. Once you've gotten her to a place of intense sensation, don't move. Hold there as long as you can so she can absorb all the pleasure that's available to her.

Make these guidelines your only moves, your only technique. It may feel like you're sailing into open water without a map, but that's okay. Let your desire be your compass. Connect to your senses and let them guide you. You've honed your skills through OM; there's nothing to do now except trust. The orgasm is there. It wants to come through. Feel your way, and everything she always knew should be available from sex will suddenly be within reach. In front of your eyes, she will bloom into the turned-on woman you have always desired.

Here's a little inspiration to help you get started.

Exercise. Slow Oral for Her

Slow Sex always begins in the same place: with desire. Feel your body, your sensations, your desire. As simply as you can, tell your partner what you want to do. Do not do anything that does not come from a true place of desire. If you want to suck her pussy, you need say nothing more than that. The truth of your desire will plant a seed within her, which will quickly grow into desire of her own.

Part One: Preparation

Consider OMing first. A woman who's been stroked will be heavy and filled with blood. She will be like a velvet cave, expanded with orgasm, surface area engorged and shimmering. Every pore, every nerve ending will be exposed, open, pulsing, and ready for your touch.

If you choose to begin this way, tell her in advance. Make her feel taken care of by safeporting her every step of the way, from the very beginning. Tell her that you intend to stroke her, but you will not give her grounding strokes at the end like you usually do. Instead, you will leave her high and full and ready. You will carefully put away all the OMing supplies while she awaits the next course.

Make every move a move of drawing her out, rather than going in and finding her. Draw her out physically and with your words: for women, there is nothing more erotic than intimate communication. Talk to her; ask her to tell you what she is feeling. And remember that there is no goal in Slow Sex; you are simply pulling the orgasm out of her one strand at a time. Let your only desire be to extend her desire; to get it to reach for you. In the process you are giving her the rare opportunity to feel the depth, weight, and power of her very own hunger. Help her welcome the experience of high sensation, so she can start to go toward it instead of pulling away. You are giving her that gift when you go slow.

Part Two: Coaxing Her Orgasm into Bloom

Speak to her. Tell her that tonight you will use your body like a magnet. You'll extract every last drop of ache and desire from her. Every part of her body will come alive; every last soft inch of tissue will be reaching and stretching toward you. Everything she normally keeps compressed and drawn in will move to the surface. You will surprise her with the enormity of what you are able to pull forth from her. It is so rare for a woman's sex to be extracted from her that most of us have never felt it. As you draw out her desire, she will get to see her sex stretch out for what may be the very first time.

If she is not already naked, help your woman take off her clothes. Go slowly; remember, for her you can never go too slowly. Linger. Show her that you care about every button, every hook, every zipper. Sit her down on the edge of the bed and kneel down in front of her. Remove her socks one at a time; help her slide her pants off. Then help her down on the bed, making sure she is comfortable and supported. While she watches you, take off your own clothes. Feel your own body warming up.

Begin with her feet. Press your thumbs into her arches, pressing and resting until you feel her really let go and exhale into the sensation. If you don't feel her relaxing, ask her to communicate her sensations to you. Ask her to tell you what it feels like in her body. Keep drawing out her sensation until you feel that she is truly ready to begin.

Take a knee in each of your hands and press each of her legs open, firmly and gently. Press for an extra moment; let her know she is handled. Feel her relax into the experience of being spread open by you. Slowly slide your hands down her calves and grip her ankles. Hold her there until you feel her relax one more level.

Slowly slide up her body, keeping yourself an inch above her. Let the tip of your cock run along her leg slightly. Once you have reached her face, look at her closely without touching her. Then lean back on your knees. Make sure you are strad-dling her but not touching her. Reach for both of her arms and spread them open. Press them down into the bed until you feel her let go.

Tips for Slow Oral for Her

Start with an OM. Prepare her body by stroking her first.

Safeport her. Tell her everything you are going to do before you do it.

Communicate. Tell her what you are feeling in your body, and ask her what she's feeling in hers.

Stay present. Be there to receive the sensations that arise throughout.

Ground her frequently. Press her body firmly but gently as you go, to ground her energy and make her feel handled.

Go even slower. Go way more slowly than you think.

Pause and feel. Stop and hold every so often.

Follow your own desire. Do what feels good in your own body and it will feel good in hers, too.

Move your face toward hers once again. Feel the heat between you. Feel the heat increase the longer you linger over her. If she moves, tell her to be still. She is not responsible for you. Put your face near her neck, under her jawline, so that your lips almost touch her tender skin. Linger there, letting a buzz build in your lips. Take tiny sips of air, again drawing some deeper part of her to the surface.

Run your fingers in a very light, circular motion over one of her nipples, taking care not to touch it. Repeat on the other side. Bring your mouth over her nipple and let the moist heat of your breath cover it, as if you were fogging up a window. Now, hover your mouth over all of her stomach and breasts, breathing against her body with a slow hot breath. Continue down her body, past her pussy, down her thighs.

Part Three: Drawing Out Her Orgasm

With one soft finger, gently skim along her inner labia. Add lubrication if that would feel good. Feel how soft her labia are, like tissue paper. Feel how, when you stroke very lightly, you can almost feel the ridges of your own fingerprints.

Bring your finger to rest just below her clit. Then softly ask her to tell you a secret. Let her know that you won't move until she tells you something confidential. Then don't move an inch until she does. As she starts talking, move your finger very, very slightly. Slowly move one millimeter closer to her clitoris without touching it directly. Get as close as you can without actually reaching it. Very, very close.

Give her tiny, soft kisses, as if your lips were swathed in gauze.

Bring your tongue down to her inner thighs. Lick the inside of each thigh as you would lick an ice cream cone that is dripping down the side. Draw the desire out of her thighs with your tongue. As her desire builds, begin to suck very slightly against her inner thigh.

Now place one hand on each of her hips and press down with firm intention and gentle pressure. As you do, let your face hover over her pussy. Feel yourself drawing out her desire. Continue to press down gently on her hips until you can feel her sinking down into the bed.

Ask her to tell you how her pussy feels. As she does, lick the valley where her inner thigh and pussy come together.

After she tells you what she feels, tell her a sensation you feel in exchange. Be specific. Describe what your cock feels like, what your chest feels like, what color, pressure, texture, and motion you are feeling inside.

Lick the outer rim of the outer labia on both sides. Lick just enough to feel the blood inside her lips moving beneath your tongue's pressure. Then, starting at her introitus, draw your tongue up the centerline of her pussy, slowly washing over her clitoris. After a few gentle strokes, take the whole of her clit into your mouth. Draw it in. Move your tongue along the bottom ridge of the clit, where her inner labia begin to separate. Move in up and down the ridge, sucking gently as you go.

Pause, and feel how her clit extends itself farther in your mouth, desiring more. Now take the whole of your mouth and engulf her clit, letting your lips relax and soften until she can't tell where they end and her own labia begin. Move the soft inside of your lips around her hood while keeping the center of your lips wrapped around her clit. Make your mouth big and soft. From time to time, pull back and exhale heat onto her clit before diving in and suckling some more.

Part Four: Going Deeper

Curve your tongue and insert it into the pocket that forms under her hood, just above her clit. There is a spot somewhere along the top ridge of the clit where you can feel a slight electrical current, like when you rub your tongue over a copper wire. Keep moving your tongue over that spot. Fuck her there, digging deeply as if you were burrowing inside her. Feel how the more attention you give it, the more the spot expands until it's pulsing under your tongue. Once it is pulsating, you know her spot is open. Wrap your mouth around the whole of her hood as you move your tongue over this spot, just above the clit.

While you are sucking her, take two fingers and slide them inside her. Feel how the blood in her skin is hot against your fingers as you do. Feel the weight of her pussy. Reach up inside her, to the spot that would be the back of her clit, and you will find a spot right there that is soft, like the top of a baby's head. Rest your fingers there. *You do not need to move.* Just press very gently. Notice how the pressure pushes her clit from behind, how it pops forward into your mouth. Suck it as if you were sucking all the juices out of it.

Feel the juices flow into your belly and down to your cock.

Begin to move your tongue in a slow rhythm that she can catch on to. If it starts to feel tight or tense, pull back and breathe. Exhale.

Ask her if she desires a climax, if she wants you to suck her until she comes. If she says yes, tell her you will be drawing her over rather than pressing her over. Gently ask her to communicate if she would like you to move faster or apply more pressure.

Then continue to push her clit slightly from behind, while sucking and moving your tongue over her. You do not need to add speed or pressure unless she asks for it. Keep sucking, but pull your tongue back on top of her clit so she can lock into you. You can create a beautiful arc where you hold her in total stillness as she comes.

As she goes over, stay present. Stay connected. Do not try to make her come; simply magnetize her orgasm toward you. Feel how there is an electrical charge running through her body. As you release the sucking, feel her body go into the familiar contractions. The longer you spend in the stillness, the more powerful the contractions will be. It will feel like her pussy is sucking your fingers up inside it, drawing you in.

As the contractions slow, move back slowly so that you can apply pressure to her body. You can apply pressure anywhere on her body, and it will ground her pussy; remember, it's all connected for a woman. Straddle her and press both hands down against her heart and chest, between her breasts. Slowly move your hands to her shoulders, and once again press down firmly. When you feel her relax, stretch out and lie on top of her until you can feel every part of her body exhale. Do not worry if she begins to cry. Wrap your arms around her so she knows you are still there.

Then, tell *her* a secret.

Slow Sex for Men

We've always thought that what men wanted was simple: sex. And of course, they do want sex. We all do. But contrary to popular mythology, sex in its traditional definition is not *all* that men want. They want climax, yes, but they also want orgasm—orgasm in its most expansive form: that state of total absorption in pleasurable sensation that all of us are looking for to nourish and hydrate a deeper part of ourselves. Men want both sides of orgasm, in other words, including the side that comes most naturally to women. Moreover, they want to plug into us, because we have access to that which they are missing.

And yet we women are frozen in a state of withholding that orgasm, not feeding our own hunger for fear of losing ground to him. For fear that he will pillage and burn the only thing we own that is really ours. We've used diversion tactics, complaints, and meanness (both subtle and overt) to keep our storehouse safe. Orgasm, we believe, is all that we have.

As a result, we are all starving.

So when we ask the question "What do men want?" the answer is simple. They want to know how to unfreeze you, because you hold the key to what they want most in life. You hold the key to their happiness.

Oh, and they want sex. That, too. But they want the kind of sex that a *woman* truly desires—the kind that turns her on, the kind she enjoys just as much as he does. So, just as I instruct the men to stroke for their own pleasure during OM, my primary instruction for women during any form of Slow Sex is to go for her own pleasure rather than his. This is easy enough to do during OM, and seems workable (if not exactly status quo) when it comes to intercourse as well. Performing oral sex on him, however, is a different issue. Though this isn't the case for every single woman, overall we've categorized the blow job as an act of self-less altruism. If we enjoy it at all, we enjoy it because it makes us feel powerful—it's one of the few ways we can consistently bring him to his knees—and also because we genuinely love him and it makes us happy to provide him with such exquisite pleasure. But using it as a reliable, even preferred path to our own get-off? Most of us have not considered it, and we wouldn't know where to begin to try.

Bringing the principles of Slow Sex to the art of oral sex is a place to begin. Strip it down, feel the sensation in your body, and follow your own desire. Here is something to get you started.

Exercise. Slow Oral for Him (aka, Cocksucking for Her Pleasure)

First, there must be desire—yours. Not the desire to please him, not the desire to get something in return, but simply the desire to feel the sensation of your mouth wrapped around him. The desire to feel the sensations that rise and fall, from your pussy to your tongue, as you stroke his cock up and down with your lips. The way his quiet moans enter your body, mixing in with your sensations until it feels like they are yours as well as his.

If you are sucking him for any other reason, do not move forward. You will only be refreezing what has become looser, more permeable, more liquid through OM. Do something else instead: have intercourse, have an OM. Save Slow Oral for another day, until the idea of sucking his cock for your own pleasure ignites a desire within you that is so powerful, so undeniable, that nothing could keep you away.

Part One: Preparation

Look at your man. See him for all of who he is—for his strength and his toughness, as well as for his vulnerability and his disappointments. Feel the love you have for him. Feel the desire you have for him. Then, if your desire is truly there, ask him gently, kindly, if he would allow you to suck his cock. Warn him that you will be doing so for your own pleasure; this will be different from oral sex he may have received in the past. Let that land with him. Give him the chance to feel the sensation of your true desire. The truth that you are doing this for *you*. The fact that you will be enjoying this as much, if not more, than he will be. He may never have felt this before; do not move too quickly.

Part Two: Tasting the Sensation of His Arousal

Ask him to take off his clothes, and take yours off as well. Go at your own pace, yet do not feel the need to linger. Have him lie down on the bed. Help him get into position; put pillows behind his knees and head. Adjust and position him. You want him to feel how you are handling him. He doesn't need to do anything. You are in control. Move him to suit your desire; follow the sensations you feel in your own body.

Allow your animal instinct to rise to the surface of your skin. Let your breasts skim his body as you move over him, feeling the electricity grow between you. He may want to adjust his own position, but that is not for him to do. If you sense him about to move, press down on him using steady, gentle pressure, holding him until he stills. Let him know he is not the one in charge. Remind him that you appreciate his help, but that you don't need it—you have this entirely under control. Touch him the way you touch something you know very well; something you own. Take possession of his body. Do not be tentative.

Tips for Slow Oral for Him

Feed your own hunger. Only perform oral sex for him if you truly have the desire to do so.

Tell him your desire. Tell him how much you want to suck his cock and how you are going to do it for your own pleasure rather than his.

Notice him. Look at him deeply before you begin.

Ground him repeatedly. Press down firmly on his body throughout so he knows you are in control.

Feel your body. Feel your own sensations as you go.

Go further. Explore his undercock, his balls, and the soft spot at the back of your own throat.

Be conscious. Stay present and aware throughout.

Feel your own desire, and take pleasure as you knead his body. Let your arousal draw out his own. Feel the way his muscle and bone rest beneath your hands. Be sure to take everything from him that you want.

Smell his skin. Inhale his scent, the way an animal tracks its prey. Draw the scent of him down into your belly, farther down into your genitals. You are taking him inside you. How does he feel there?

Put your ear to his belly. Listen to the sounds of him. Go inside him in this way; see how far inside him your attention can penetrate. Listen to the way his body thumps and roars. Feel the aliveness inside him, how every part of him is in motion.

Now press down on his chest firmly. See if you can push with your own inner body, the invisible one. Push as if you are pushing yourself into him. As if you can see in, through his skin and into his chest. Then rest there. Be still inside him. Then allow your body to slide down along his, the way you would rub your body along silk sheets.

Part Three: Drawing Out His Orgasm

Gently rub your cheeks and face inside his legs. Feel how being near his cock electrifies you. Feel every sensation as you inch closer and closer. Absorb each sensation as if you were digesting it. Feel it spread out to your extremities, nourishing every cell of your body in the process.

When the sensations of desire become too much to bear, you are ready. Take him in your hands.

Look at his cock. Study it carefully. Notice the coloring along the rim, the way a vein pulses along the shaft. Feel the tenderness of this most tender organ. How when it is not yet completely hard, it is almost like a small animal. Feel its heat radiating into the skin of your hands. If he moves his hips to diminish the sensation your attention generates in him, use one hand to firmly press his hip back into the bed. Remind him that he is not in charge. Allow the heat of his cock to once again penetrate your skin.

Imagine what it will taste like. Then feel your own body. Feel your own genitals and lips, how they may swell at the thought. Feel your pussy and notice any sensation there. Is there heat, or tingling, or a desire to pull up to hold on to sensation? Try pushing out through your perineum, as if to clear anything stuck or frozen inside you. Then return your attention to his cock.

Move one hand beneath his balls, simply for the pleasure of feeling them in your hands. You are not touching him for any reason other than to take your own pleasure. He may start to rock and moan; do not be distracted. Feel his balls, how they seem to move slightly in your hand, how they are out of his volition. Then feel the firm undercock beneath them. Gently press into it, massaging it. Feel how when you press it, the shaft of his cock moves in your hand. Begin to rock his cock with both hands, back and forth, as if you were gently shimmying the bottom cock loose. Feel how both parts of him swell in unison.

Now is the moment for you to free your own desire. Free it. Then free it even more. Allow your desire to rise up like a wave; imagine that your deepest hunger is about to be fed. You can feel it deep in your stomach, all the way down to your genitals. Now imagine what it would feel like to have something warm and soft and electric touching that deep spot inside you. Feel your hunger for it, and imagine it being filled.

When you are ready, bring your mouth to his cock. Brush your lips with the head of it. Take a tiny taste like a sip, touching your tongue lightly. Taste him. Give tiny kisses, the way you would kiss a baby's head—the kind of kisses that make you feel better in the giving. When you are ready, wrap your lips around the tip, making sure not to let your teeth graze his shaft. Relax your lips as much as you can—it is possible to do with practice. Hold his cock at the base with one hand, your fingers wrapped around it in the shape of an "o." Use the other hand to push upward from the undercock, beneath his balls. Allow yourself to suck his head gently, wetting it with your saliva.

Move slowly. Take everything you can from his body; pull him into you. Draw his cock over your tongue. Feel the way it feels to brush him over your taste buds. Flick your tongue along the apex, that "v" at the front of his head. Let your tongue find that groove. When you are ready for a different sensation, slide your tongue down the vein that runs along the shaft. Feel how it has a kind of buoyancy, how it bulges on either side of where your tongue compresses. Taste him all the way down.

Only once you have taken all the pleasure you can from licking and sucking him, take his cock into your mouth. Take in as much as fits comfortably. Let it rest there in your mouth, as if letting a piece of chocolate melt on your tongue. Slowly slide it farther into your mouth, toward the back of your throat.

There is a secret I will share with you. At the back of your throat, there is a soft and fleshy point where you can access intensely pleasurable sensation. Most women never discover it, because it requires you to slide him past your gag reflex. Go slowly, and relax. You are on a mission of discovery. See if you can slide him all the way back until you can gently tap his cock against the soft spot there. If you make it, feel how it causes contractions in your throat. Relax into them. Feel how they can be as pleasurable as the contractions in your pussy when he strokes you. Allow your throat to soften and wrap around his cock as you stroke your soft spot with the tip of it. Feel how it seems to send shock waves down to your pussy and back up again. Feel how your mouth begins to feel like an extension of your pussy.

Slowly pull him out of your mouth. Feel the pleasure of it. As you pull his cock out of your throat apply a slight sucking, so you are pulling him gently in opposite directions. Feel how when that tension in your throat relaxes, it spreads out in waves through the rest of your body. Then pull him back into your throat, and notice how all of you seems to tighten and squeeze around him. Let your whole being fold around him in this way. Gather all your attention and place it on his cock in your mouth.

If you find yourself feeling emotional, don't hold back. Let it all flow. Feel how sexy it is to let go of all decorum, to feed your hunger first before trying to look good.

Part Four: Going Deeper

Feel your own body and the energy of orgasm running through it. Do you have a desire to bring him to climax? If so, keep running him in and out of your mouth, using your hands as an extension of your mouth. With your tongue, press against the front of his cock as you run up and down. Allow your tongue to hit his apex every time you come up.

You will feel him swell in your mouth as he prepares to go over. Check in with your desire. Do you have a hunger to take his come in your belly? If so, slide him back into your throat and milk the climax out of him. If not, take care of the final touches with your hands.

Stay conscious and present as he goes over. Feel him contract in your mouth or your hands. Move slowly. Once he is finished, squeeze him firmly. Hold him there. Just as when he grounds you after an OM, he can take more pressure than you probably expect. Hold him until you feel a landing in his body or your own; until it feels like something has completely exhaled.

Get up and wet a towel with warm water. Squeeze it out and wrap it around his cock. Clean him up sweetly, using your attention to wipe him slowly, carefully, intimately. Dry him off with a dry towel. Take your time here. You're grounding his body and your own, and integrating the orgasmic experience the two of you had together.

Slow Intercourse

Intercourse is the centerpiece, the glorious beating heart of our sexual universe. It calls forth the best of everything we have: body, soul, flesh, desire. But because it shines so brightly, it can't help but draw out our shadow as well. Our shame and self-consciousness, our insecurities and most deeply rooted fears.

Intercourse is the spark that sets all life in motion; quite literally, it's the beginning of everything. Everything except Slow Sex, as you may have noticed. In this world, intercourse comes at the end, after we've stripped down and thawed out and learned how to feel and learned how to open. It comes after we've taken the time to listen and feel and understand one another. Because its very centrality, its primacy within the sexual landscape, means it magnetizes our most stubborn and complicated habits. We have been carrying around so many *very big ideas* about it, and for so long—since we were ten or twelve or sixteen years old—that it takes quite a bit of OM-level unlearning before we can trust ourselves to drop down into its warm embrace without the armor of expectation, judgment, and self-criticism.

But it can be done. All it takes is subtracting anything extra, letting sensation chart your course, and staying open to whatever comes up along the way. And while sex does not take well to a recipe, I've discovered over the years that it's perfectly happy to receive a little nudge in the right direction. So here I offer you, for inspiration rather than replication, a Slow Sex guide for Slow...*Sex*.

Exercise. Slow Intercourse

We begin, as always, with desire. Many reasons come to mind for having sex, some of them desire-based and others not. But here, today, let it be for desire. Which sensations of desire can you feel in your body? Do they feel warm, glowing, rising? Do they feel sticky, tingly, aching? Can you feel your partner's desire, using your own senses as a thermometer? Does your partner's desire draw you in, immerse you? Or does it repel you, even slightly, like the wrong side of a magnet? Feel the desire to merge, the intimate dance that is rising between you. You do not need to add anything to it. Simply take the time to feel the sensations in your body before you begin.

Part One: Preparation

Carefully choose the location where you are going to fuck, making sure it feels lush and sexy, a safe haven, a nest where your desire can come out of its shell unharmed. Bring in pillows or blankets if you want a soft landing. Or strip down to the bare sensation of the two of you, on a sheet, on the bed.

Leave the lights on. Not glaring, not harsh, but soft and revealing. Let your partner see every part of you, draw in every nutrient you have to offer.

Help your partner remove their clothes. Get down on your knees in front of them; help them remove each sock; slide their pants to the floor. Then let them help you with yours, carefully unbuckling your belt, slowly unzipping your jeans, sweater over the head, hair tousled and tangled and beautiful.

Prepare one another, your naked bodies warming up with every touch. Turn on your senses—your feeling and tasting, listening and smelling. Knead each other; taste one another's skin. Feel your partner's body under your hands; see if you can run your fingertips over every part of her body before you ever lie down. What does he taste like? Does she smell like an animal, gamey and ripe, or like sunlight, sweet and salty at the same time?

Feel the negotiations your bodies are making. Use your whole bodies. Stretch and fold into each other. Feel the engine revving inside you; feel the urge to mount and scratch the itch that brought you to this place. Sink your teeth into your partner's flesh, digging and then resting. Let him feel the danger of your deepest hunger, rising to the surface. Notice the moments of shyness or surges of power. Pay attention. You are getting into relationship not just with your partner, but with the orgasm that is already rising between you.

Tips for Slow Intercourse

Feel your desire. Experience the rising turn-on and talk about it with your partner.

Choose the right location. Create a space that matches the kind of sex you want to have.

Leave the lights on. Sex is not something to keep in the dark.

Undress together. Savor the revelation of your partner's body, moment by moment.

Go slowly. Feel, communicate, and explore, knowing and letting the hunger build.

> **Shift stroke.** Feel deeply and change your stroke when sensation begins to decrease.
> **Feel the orgasm.** Speak your sensations as orgasm builds, peaks, and crests between you.
> **Tell one another what you desire.** Feel the vibration in your throat as the sound exits. Feel how good it is to use your voice, to reveal yourself.

Feel all the different ways your bodies might come together. Do you want to sit atop him, pressing with your hands down hard into his chest, letting your hair fall on his face? Or do you want to lie back, a slight whimper in your throat as he takes you? Do you want to lie side-by-side, your legs wrapped around him, your breasts pressed against him so not even a slip of tissue-light paper could come between you? Do you want to hold his hands back over his head and feel him as a captive? Let out your bad and dangerous desires—the ones that normally only whisper to you through fantasy. This is the time when everything can come out and play.

Part Two: Heavier Strokes

Kiss him. Let your saliva mix and mingle, then glide your lips across hers so lightly. Feel how the electricity grows when you do. Feel the pull to press harder. Then don't. Slide your tongue along the outline of his lips. Feel the tender inside, the little bumps and grooves. Feel the underside of your tongue on the inside of her lip and how naked it feels. Push his mouth open with yours. Run your tongue along the roof of it.

Apply lube to your partner's genitals, until both of you are slick and smooth. Stroke one another gently. Move your whole body in unison with the stroke. Keep cock and pussy close together, but not yet touching. Feel the heat between them, how they are already connected. Feel the texture of your partner's most sensitive spot beneath your fingers. Knead it gently.

When the time is right for entry, you will feel it in your body.

Hand her the condom and let her unwrap it and roll it over you.

Take the head of his cock into your pussy. Just the tip. Feel the way a sort of suction builds, the way her pussy reaches up to swallow more, the way his cock desires to dive farther inside her. Feel how hard it is to pull it back out, and do it anyway. Pause for a moment and feel the tension between having and wanting. Let the tension build as the head of his cock catches on the rim of her entrance. Feel how your genitals feel sealed to one another. You are ready.

Now, slowly slide his cock farther into your pussy, feeling as each of your ridges pass over one another. Allow your labia to spread open and your clitoris to press down on his pubic bone. Grind together and feel the tension building. Feel your soft flesh spreading over his cock like honey.

Pause and feel the connections throughout your body. Continue to move her clit over your pubic bone in a slight rocking motion. See if you can tap the back of her clit with the head of your cock. She will feel a rush from the back to the front—like a current that surges back and forth.

Pull him to the very tip again and begin with shallow strokes. Create a rhythm: ten shallow strokes and then slide down hard. Ten shallow strokes and then slide down hard. Allow your pussy to shake, to quiver against his cock. Push out, toward each other. Feel how his cock is getting stroked by the back of your clit, from the inside.

Whenever you sense that you have hit a peak of sensation—

that the next movement will be less sensational than the last—the time has come to shift stroke. Consciously exhale. Breath cleans the palate, prepares you for the next peak. Rest there, connected with your partner. Notice how she is different, already, from the one you lay down with.

Now feel again the seal between cock and pussy. Feel the point of contact between the interior clit—just behind the exterior clit—and the head of his cock, how they feel suctioned together. Use his cock as a plunger against that spot; let his cock suck it open. When it opens, she will feel a quiet pop. It is like the pop of a bottle of sparkling water opening. She will feel as if bubbles were overflowing into the next layer of her pussy. Her lower abdomen will feel full, and at the same time alive. He will feel it as if he has popped through to a new place, and that place is filled with something thick and viscous.

Part Three: The Evolution of Intercourse

This is the point where most people end, where both partners go for climax and the experience is over. But that is only one choice. For here, from this place of deepest connection, the other side of orgasm becomes available. Very few take the time to access it, or even realize it is there. It is as different from "regular" sex as day is from night. It is a kind of gateway that opens to a whole new plateau, a whole new level of pleasurable sensation.

To access this orgasmic state, simply feel what is happening between you.

Feel how every last cell of your body feels hydrated and full—how very little movement is required to garner much sensation. Your whole body may tremble in moving only a quarter of an inch. Feel the alive stillness, how it is empty and yet has substance. Feel how you are both being held inside a mutual orgasm rather than trying to arrive at it as a destination.

It is here where the instructions fall away. All we do is follow our sensations toward what feels good. What feels good tends to be quite slow, imbued with a sense of depth and sensation. Every movement is revelatory. There is a heartrending poignancy to each gesture. A kiss at this point feels fresh and new, as if you have never felt the wonder of lips touching your own. This is where you may feel yourself in the slow animal dance of sniffing and circling. You may want to mount your partner; you may want to pull away. You may simply want to explore the sensation of having him inside you. He will be out of the ejaculation zone, and therefore may soften. Feel that softening; let it melt both your hearts. There is nothing right or wrong to do here.

Or maybe you both do want to go over. Ask your partner: Do you want to go further? Are you satiated? Feel the response. If you decide to go for climax, stay connected as you go over. You may want to speak. You may want to kiss. You may want to make eye contact. Whatever you do, stay with one another through all the contractions. Drink in the physicality of it, the rawness, the realness, the saturation. Feel the rise and fall of the orgasm that was born between you in this experience, and watch as love for your partner naturally fills your heart.

Slow Sex gives you access to sex as it was meant to be—as you suspected it could be, as you hoped it might be. It's like the power turns on. Whereas before you had to wind your clock manually, now the hands move of their own accord. Sex that was a physical act requiring effort now seems to run on its own fuel. That fuel is turn-on. When you truly get turned on, you find that more energy, more sensation, and more connection are available during sex.

More turn-on during sex means more turn-on everywhere else, too. Turn-on is the energy of life, of flow, of being carried by a force greater than yourself. And the way we access it is simple: we consciously engage our own desire. In sex, yes, but in every other area of our lives as well. Cultivating turn-on is how we extend the orgasmic experience beyond the bounds of what we thought was possible, how we become orgasmic not only in the bedroom but also in life itself. And how to create more of it in your life is the final lesson I teach to my Slow Sex students: the lesson of the next chapter, The Four-Month Orgasm.

Chapter Nine

The Four-Month Orgasm

I love men. I want them to have everything they desire. I want them to feel connected, seen, and understood. Yet, in order for that to happen, men need women. Women to show them what possibilities emerge when they are willing to let go of control. Women to show them what unconditional appreciation looks like, what turn-on feels like, what intimacy feels like. Women who are ignited. Women who are orgasmic.

So if I'm completely honest, I didn't write this book for men. I wrote it for women—for myself, for my friends, for the women I see every day in the work I do. These are spectacular women, women whose true power could light New York City. Women whose beauty could bring you to your knees.

Women who have no idea how much power they actually have. Women who spend a lot of energy making themselves into the shape of a good woman, because that's the only thing they've ever learned how to do.

Women who desire to feel plugged in and connected, who know that deeper connection has to be possible.

In other words, women who want to be unfailingly orgasmic—orgasmic every single moment of every single day.

I don't think I have to tell you that very few women are living life this way. We've barely let ourselves dare to hope that this kind of life exists, much less tried to figure out how to get one for ourselves. The irony is that this is the very sort of life we are all meant to be living, but few of us know how to access it. Just as I discovered that afternoon in the kitchen with Uncle Bob, we have never really learned how to taste a tomato. How to be present and aware as we bite into it, and then to actually feel—and be able to name—the sensation of *sour-electric-hydrated* as it washes across the tongue. To feel all the joy and plea-sure available in that bite, to integrate it into our bodies so it becomes fuel for the journey. We are born connected to a universal grid of everyday magic; it comes with the pack-age of life. Our job is simply to plug into it. One easy way to plug into the magic is through Orgasmic Meditation.

The magic, of course, *is* orgasm. Orgasm in the expanded sense—the orgasm we feel coming through us when we OM, but which we can feel in every minute of every day if we are attuned to it. Plugging into this kind of orgasm comes more naturally to women, and as such it is our responsibility to bring it into the world, for everyone else—including our men—to enjoy. The problem is, we don't treat our orgasm as we should: like a precious natural resource. As women, we either ignore it or spend our time trying to make it into something more than what it already is. We turn our attention toward action, actively pursuing climax and positioning and technique, when the channel that comes more naturally to us is reception. Reception means opening to whatever comes through us, receiving and welcoming our genuine orgasm, regardless of whether it meets our expectations or fits into a particular mold. Reception is listening to our orgasm like an artist would, plunging our roots deep into it so we can be hydrated. We spend a lot of time searching for orgasm, striving for it, sending out a missing persons alert for it, when in truth it's been right in front of us the entire time. If we don't recognize the oasis of our orgasm, how can we drink from it? Is it any wonder that we—men and women alike—are living in a desert?

So as you can see, when I say that you should OM every day, there's a lot at stake.

Connecting to this orgasm is the deeper purpose of OM. OM holds both of us, stroker and receiver alike, in a state of receptive openness for at least fifteen minutes a day. It gives us an easy way to marinate in the sensations that are already coming through our bodies so they can nourish us. Even if we choose to spend the rest of the day in a state of action—driving, pursuing, and directing our experience— for these fifteen minutes, we agree to do the opposite. We OM. We connect, we plug back in, and we go deeply wherever the orgasm wants to lead us.

The orgasm we plug into when we OM has no limitations, no boundaries. It is a cup that is never empty, a resource that constantly renews itself. This is the message I try to convey to my students at the beginning of the OM workshop, that at the end of the course they'll have all the tools they need to experience a four-month orgasm. What I really mean is that by the end of the class, they'll know everything they need to know in order to have a *lifelong* orgasm—to live orgasmically, in every moment.

I actually say the "four-month" part because it's more believable.

The key to having a lifelong orgasm is not OM, exactly. OM is just the rehearsal; it's where we learn the music, build the muscle memory, develop the habits that will support us when we get out onstage. It's where we practice for the main performance: life. Life, including "regular" sex, and male-female relationship, and everything else we do. The habits we form through OM—habits of receptivity, appreciation, awareness, true intimacy—are 180 degrees opposite from the habits that rule our conventional world. So learning to make them our default settings takes practice. It takes great attention and precision to choose subtraction— simplicity—in a culture that hawks addition at every turn. It takes repetition to learn how to pay attention enough to feel sensation in the body, to experience turn-on as it rises, crests, and carries us. And it takes a practiced willingness to feel what you want and then be vulnerable, intimate, and open enough to ask for it, come what may.

"What drew me in about OM is that it's a microcosm for life. Every single thing you experience during that fifteen-minute session is going to come up again when you get up and go about your day. Every moment of joy, every sensation in your body, every disappointment, every success. It's all there. Even the things that you usually ignore—they're the first things that come up in your practice. It's a tremendous relief to have those things be seen and to engage them on a conscious level, because there's nowhere to hide. OM becomes a practice not just for sex, but for your whole life." —Jonathan, 38

It takes all those things, yes, but it takes one thing more. When it gets down to it, there must be a willingness to change your navigation device. We tend to navigate our lives using signposts set up for us by the world—norms, expectations, shoulds, and should nots. If you want a lifelong orgasm, you have to let go of the comfort of being told what to do by the outside world and start looking for direction within. You have to start charting your own course, using your own compass. That compass is your own desire.

Using Desire as a Compass

The concept of using desire as a compass takes a little getting used to. I generally hear two responses when I start talking about it in class. On the one hand—and more often from women—they believe they don't have enough desire to begin with. What they do have is buried so deeply they can't even find it; how are they supposed to use it as a compass? The second argument—more often from men— is that if they followed their desire all the time, they would never get any work done. All they'd be doing would be having sex.

Both are valid concerns, and both clear up with a bit of recalibration—recalibration that comes naturally as a part of Orgasmic Meditation. First, the stroke is designed to bring hidden desire to the surface. It coaxes the truth out, little by little, until it becomes impossible not to see that what you actually want is to kiss your stroker, or to find a new job, or to spend more time with your children. During the practice you're building the habit of watching the sensations in your body, in effect honing your desire-detection instrument. In the same way, asking for the stroke you want during OM increases your capacity to be more open and vulnerable when it comes to putting your desires out into the world. After OMing for a while, most people discover they are much more comfortable asking for what they want in their lives at large.

You are not alone in your fear that if you use your desire as a compass your life will devolve into barbaric hedonism. Most of us have created deep patterns of denying ourselves what we want because we believe that our desire is a bottomless pit. If we dare begin to feed our hunger, to approve of it, we'll be letting a wild animal out of a cage. Soon, this animal will be terrorizing the whole village, burning and pillaging and, in its spare time, having a whole lot of sex.

In truth, the reawakening of desire is usually a lot quieter. I remember when I first really allowed myself to use desire as my compass. I was living in a community of OM practitioners, where we were encouraged to OM as often as we liked. When I was getting ready to move in, my desire for OM was so great that the thought crossed my mind: what if moving in cost me my job? How would I make it to work when all I'd want to be doing was OMing? Sure enough, as soon as I moved in and gave my desire permission to roam, I went through an extended period where OM was the only thing I wanted to do. But somehow, I still managed to show up for work every day. Turns out that in addition to my desire for OM, I had a desire to keep a roof over my head and food in my belly. Go figure.

And as insatiable as my desire for OM felt at the beginning, there was a moment where things changed. After several months of a whole lot of OM, I remember my partner asking me if I wanted to practice. I checked in with my internal compass, and to my surprise, I didn't have the desire to OM. My first response was fear.

"I think I lost my desire!" I said in panic to my teacher.

"Did it ever occur to you," she asked, "that you might have just gotten full?"

The thought had never crossed my mind. My hunger had been an insatiable beast yearning to be fed for as long as I could remember. Like a good girl, I had denied it everything it was asking for, secretly hoping it would starve to death. Now, through OM, I had started to feed it a little each day. Voracious at first, over time and with a consistent diet, the desire became less and less needy, less and less hungry. Then one day, just like that, it was full. Deliciously, powerfully, incredibly full.

That fullness is the key to lifelong orgasm. It paves the way for extending out to others, others who desperately need to see that fullness is possible in order to begin looking for it themselves. But we only get full when we are willing to follow our desire and feed the hunger within, consistently and over a long period of time. Feeding our desire, paying attention to it, is why we OM. When we OM, we drop down into the ocean of desire in a way we rarely take the time to do otherwise. We marinate in our own sensations for fifteen minutes, letting our desire rise up and then seep back down into our deepest places. Desire is sweetness; it is the elixir of life. It inspires, lubricates, satisfies, and satiates. Desire is the artist's muse. When my students start to spend time in her company, they are inspired.

Desire is also our native wisdom, our true north. It points us in the direction we are meant to go—the place where the most sensation will be found. The more sensation, the more enjoyment. The more enjoyment, the happier we are. Do a little bit of arithmetic, and desire begins to look like the road to happiness.

This shouldn't be a surprise when you take the time to look at the world we live in. A brief investigation reveals that our universe is entirely desire-based. Desire keeps our world running; it's the fuel of life. It's what draws the bee toward the flower, what keeps the planet populated with flora, fauna, and—well, human beings. Desire is the natural order of things, the evolutionary driver. It's how traits that will serve the species get integrated into the fabric of the whole. It's what compels us to up our game as a species. Every living thing follows its implicit impulse and becomes a better and better version of itself in the process.

Except us.

Somewhere along the way, we humans took a different road. We veered off from the evolutionary path. By contrast to all the other species with whom we share our world, we developed the capacity for self-reflection; we saw that it is even *possible* to curb desire. The bee can't ponder whether it has "too much" desire for nectar and then set New Year's resolutions, after all. We humans are the only ones who have the capacity for discernment, for choosing which desires to follow and which to repress.

Which, from the point of view of society, may not seem like such a bad thing. If everyone followed their individual desires, we assume, the world would be bedlam. There would be no rules, no right and wrong. We'd each be chasing every impulse we had, regardless of how it might affect others. This assumption, I can now say from experience, is a fallacy of the hungry. When we are repressing our desires, telling them to go to bed without dinner, they start to get a little cranky. We have all assumed that if we let these cranky little beasts run wild, they'd soon run us straight into the ground. And maybe there would be a period of mayhem (maybe not), but what I can say from my own experience is that one day, equilibrium would be reached. If we committed to following our desires, hunger would no longer be a problem. Just look at the way the natural world works; when each species follows its desires, you don't get a war zone—you get an *ecosystem*. Each does its part within the greater whole, and the result is coopera- tion, co-evolution, and harmony. Soon, what you have is a mature, deep-rooted forest.

Killing our desire out of fear keeps us hungry, irritable, and rooted in shallow soil. We may feel a sense of secu- rity, of staying in society's good graces, but we don't expe- rience aliveness. We don't get nourishment, we don't get hydration. We don't get great sex, great art, or great poetry. "Great" can only come through when we stop setting our compass toward "good." Figure that piece out, and you'll start to see turn-on everywhere you look.

Turning On

If there's anything I've learned over many years of prac- ticing Slow Sex, it's that fighting against desire gets you nowhere. Long ago, I agreed to go wherever desire took me, and the reward I've gotten in return is the opportunity to live a turned-on life. When we decide to fuel our life with desire rather than fear, it's like switching tanks. It's the dif- ference between running on fossil fuel versus solar power. When we choose solar, we are no longer forced to mine our own resources in order to get where we're going. What fuels us now is the endless resource of turn-on. We move from the "action" channel to the "receiving" channel—from a place of accomplishing things by *doing* to a place of accomplishing things simply by *receiving*. This is the glory of the desire-based life: things become easy; synchronicities abound; and everything you desire comes your way almost effortlessly.

Turn-on is available everywhere, at all times—you need only tune in to your desire to access it. When you pay attention to your desire, you learn what brings you enjoyment. And the natural outcome of enjoyment is turn-on. When you follow where your desire takes you, you can't help but be carried away by turn-on. That's why we come back to activities we love again and again. We feel nourished by our own enjoyment, by the opportunity to sink our roots deeply into something and receive turn-on in return.

When we start living with desire as our compass, everything begins to change. We start to see all the ways in which our habits are getting in the way of actually living. All the rules we've been taught—fake it till you make it, win at any cost, suck it up, never give up—are effective if you want to get ahead in the world at the cost of any chance at true happiness. But the world of enjoyment has an entirely different set of rules: Increase attention rather than pressure. Fill up before you extend outward. Follow your desire until turn-on flows. If it feels like work, change the stroke. When in doubt, play.

Such a switch requires nothing less than a reworking of your entire relationship to your own desire. Taking desire from the cranky passenger in the backseat and inviting it to take the wheel. And—this is important—*to drive wherever it wants to go.* And by "wherever," I mean anywhere, anytime. With the promise that you will hang on for the ride, regardless of where your desire takes you.

It's a big leap, to voluntarily surrender control and let your desire forge the path instead of your "appropriate" mind. It's the leap of a lifetime, in fact. But until you're willing to take this leap, you are not truly living. For this is the leap *into life*, into your own life, your little life, the one you were handed on your way in and asked to take care of for seventy or ninety years. And where has it been all this time? Hidden in a closet? Stuffed in the trunk? The time has come to bring that golden gift out into the world. To set it on a green grassy hillside and give it the space to relearn how to play. I say "relearn," because it already knows. Our desire comes fully equipped with all the information it needs to do its part, we only have to stop trying to control it so very much.

Orgasmic Meditation is about finding our way back toward our desire, the piece that truly knows, so we can start to lead with it. The good news is that once we agree to let desire be our primary orientation, turn-on does the rest. It's as if life carries us along, opening all the right doors and directing us toward our true purpose. That's not to say that every stroke is guaranteed to be pleasurable from there on out—it won't be. Life is full of both upstrokes and downstrokes, strokes that are pleasurable and strokes that are not. What we learn instead is that contrary to our previous belief, there is turn-on available regardless of the stroke. We can get off on the downs just as well as the ups, sometimes even more so. And when we stop holding a preference for one stroke over another, we have access to the greatest commodity available in life: freedom.

Getting Off on Any Stroke

When we begin to OM, we explore all the different strokes that are possible—up, down, light, heavy, and more. Inevitably, we end up developing certain preferences: "I like upstrokes best." "I like to start softly and build to firmer re." We learn to feel our own desire and start getting rtable asking for what we want from our partner, is is an important stage in our practice. There comes , however, when we have gotten comfortable asking stroke we crave, and we never want anything *but* that stroke. Sooner or later, we feel like we can't get off without that particular stroke, like it is the only stroke that will ever make us happy.

In OM that may be fine; we can theoretically always ask for our stroker to shift and give us what we want. Life at large is a different story. In our world, we are presented with all sorts of different strokes, and we don't always get to choose which one is coming our way. One day it seems we're getting everything we want. We feel like we're golden and can do no wrong. Other days we feel like the whole world is against us and nothing is going right. We tend to have a preference for the good day, the "upstroke." We do everything we can to protect ourselves from the downstroke of the bad day. Which would be an okay idea, except that it never works. The downstroke comes, whether we resist it or not. In the process of trying to protect ourselves from the strokes we object to, we end up expending a lot of energy and not getting very far.

One of the most incredible opportunities in OM is the fact that it is a microcosm of this dynamic. Some days our partner is a master stroker and is getting us just right, and other days he's an ape-man who we never should have married in the first place. One day we love the stroke he's giving us, and the next we wish the OM was over before it even begins. Rather than being a problem, the latter can be an opportunity, that is, an opportunity to play with the possibility of getting off on any stroke at all, whether it's the one you prefer or not. The stakes are lower during an OM than they are in life. Once you know that you *could* ask your partner to shift stroke and give you something more pleasurable, you have the freedom to wait a few strokes before asking. Discover what it feels like to hold in a stroke that may not be your favorite, and see whether you could get off on it anyway. This knowledge—that no matter which stroke is coming your way, you can draw enjoyment from it—is the equivalent of learning how to say "yes" to life.

Exercise. Feeling the Sensation of "Yes"

Just saying the word "yes" has a physical impact. This short exercise is meant to help you familiarize yourself with the feeling of "yes" in your own body.

You will need a quiet spot, about ten minutes, and your journal for this exercise.

Step One. Sit comfortably, take a few deep breaths, and feel for the sensations in your body until you are sure you've set down your anchor. This exercise requires you to feel what is going on in your body, so take as long as you need to in order to get in touch with your sensations.

Step Two. Once you are anchored in sensation, repeat the word "yes" out loud several times. Say "yes, yes, yes, yes, yes." Notice what sensations it brings up for you. Where do you feel it in your body? Describe what it feels like—its texture, motion, speed, color, and pressure. Say "yes, yes, yes" a few more times if necessary until you have locked the sensations of that word into your memory.

Step Three. Take a few more breaths, and settle in once again. This time, say "no, no, no, no, no" out loud. Notice where the "no" lands in your body. Where do you feel it? What is the texture, motion, speed, color, and pressure of the word "no"? How does it compare to the word "yes"?

Step Four. Write for a few minutes in your journal about the difference between saying yes and saying no. Be sure to record all of the sensations you can remember. This exercise is simple but powerful—don't forget to record your first impressions. Write about two recent experiences: one where you said yes and one where you said no. How might these experiences have been different if you had gone the other way? What feelings come up at the thought of saying yes to everything? Fear, excitement, disbelief, liberation?

For most of us, the experience of saying yes has a naturally open quality. Regardless of the particular texture and color and motion it brings up in an individual, there is a feeling that the body wants to open wider and become more transparent when we say yes. Oftentimes, students report an opposite response to the word "no." There may be a feeling of contraction, of closing up shop, of clenching.

Staying open and aware—saying yes—is the key to getting off on any stroke, whether in OM or in life. Saying yes is the key to the freedom we were just talking about. When we let go of our preference for any one particular experience, suddenly a whole world of opportunity presents itself. We are not only more able to enjoy the upstrokes, but we can also start to investigate what nourishment might be available from the downstrokes as well. Lo and behold, we see that there is rich, earthy, sexy sensation to be drawn out of even the stroke we didn't think we wanted. In fact, it turns out there are certain experiences we actually *desire*, but which we never before allowed ourselves to have because they didn't come in the package of our preferred stroke. By learning how to say yes to whatever is presented to us, we go one step further toward following our desire— and toward living the turned-on life we truly crave.

Exercise. Getting Off on Every Stroke OM

This is a great practice to try over the course of several OMs in a row. That way you are almost guaranteed to experience some of the strokes you prefer and some that you would ordinarily resist. The goal here is to research whether it's possible to get off on even the strokes that don't meet your standard preferences. Practicing it several times over the course of a week will ensure you'll have the opportunity to say yes to a full range of strokes.

You will need all of your OMing supplies, your partner, about half an hour, and your journal.

Step One. Prepare for an OM as you usually would with your partner. If you are the stroker, begin stroking your partner. Stroke for your own pleasure; which way do you want the stroke to go? How fast or slow, heavy or light do you want it? Do not ask your partner for feedback, just stroke her clit to generate the most possible sensation in your own body.

Step Two. If you are the receiver, feel the stroke. Notice whether the stroke he is giving you feels pleasurable or not.

Step Three. As the receiver, say "yes," out loud, to every stroke. Throughout the OM, let "yes" be your moan, your vocalization.

Notice how saying yes over and over affects the sensation you are feeling in your body. Pay particular attention to what it feels like to say yes to a stroke you would normally object to. Does saying yes change your experience of that stroke? What does it feel like to say yes to the light, tickling tease? What about the grinding, piercing, nerve-jangling stroke? Continue to say yes, out loud, to every stroke.

Step Four. Reset your OMing timer for five minutes, and both partners write in your journals about the experience. Overall, did you notice anything different about this OM as opposed to a regular OM? What did you like? What didn't you like? If you were the stroker, how did it feel to stroke purely for your own pleasure—while hearing your partner say "yes" to every stroke? Record any emotions or unusual sensations that came up for you. If you were the receiver, what was it like to hold every stroke, without preference? What sensations did you feel in your body when you said yes? Both partners, if you think about saying yes to every stroke you get in life, does that feel like something you'd want to do? Why or why not?

Saying yes to any stroke is the work of a lifetime. Learning to follow your desire is a good start. What you'll discover is that the hardest part of using your desire as a compass is not a lack of desire, nor is it too much desire. It's that, in a world that is calling us to do everything but listen to our inner knowing, our own compass, desire can be very easy to forget. Forgetting, as it turns out, is the only thing between us and the lifelong orgasm we are looking for. Because when we can remember to follow our desire with every step—and to say yes to whatever we meet along the way—orgasm becomes effortless. It becomes the water we're swimming in.

I was a bit of an overachiever when I started to OM, and one day I asked my teacher what was the longest orgasm you could have.

"I don't know," he said. "How long can you remember to follow your desire?"

It was, it turned out, up to me.

At the time, I could remember to follow my desire for about thirty seconds, tops. Then something would go wrong—I'd get disappointed with a boyfriend, or I wouldn't get a job I'd really wanted—and suddenly it was like my balloon of orgasm would deflate. I had a friend at the time who seemed to be able to sustain that orgasmic state for much longer than I could, naturally saying yes to whatever came her way. I marveled at how turned on she always seemed to be. So one day I asked her how it was that she was able to hold on to the sense of expansiveness that seemed to slip out of my hands so easily.

"I remember to remember," she said simply.

If there's anything I wish for you, it is that you remember to remember. Remember that you don't have to add anything to your sex or your life—orgasm knows how to take care of itself. Remember to pay attention to the sensation in your body; it is the secret entry into the world of turn-on. And remember to always follow your desire. Use it as a compass; it will guide you toward the sustainable happiness, richness, and satisfaction you're looking for—in sex, in your relationships, and in your life as a whole.

And when in doubt, remember to OM. Because if there's one thing I know, it's that everything we desire is just waiting for us to draw it out. When you agree to make room in your busy life for fifteen minutes of intimate connection, it's like being willing to stand in the kitchen without a recipe.

In that one act, you become an artist; you let go and let life reveal itself. And what I can promise is this: stroke by stroke, all the joy and pleasure and intimacy and nourishment you could ever want from sex—and life—can't help but rise up to meet you.

Appendix: OM for Him

Besides the obvious difference, male stroking is a lot like traditional OMing. A man lies down and a woman (or another man) strokes the shaft of his penis for fifteen minutes. The man may or may not climax, but climax is not the goal. The goal is simply to experience the stroke, whether you are giving it or receiving it. In other words, just like regular OM, the foundation of male stroking is letting go of any expectations. Strip it down. Experience the stroke each time as if it were the first time. Pay attention to your sensations, and share them with your partner. Finally, make contact with the desire that lies just beneath the surface, and allow it to be brought out, stroke by stroke.

Getting Ready

Prepare for the OM as outlined in chapter 3. First, ask your partner to OM with you, making sure it is clear that you are suggesting a male-stroking OM in particular. If you are the stroker, carefully set up the OMing nest. You will need the same supplies as usual: pillows, a hand towel, lube, and a timer.

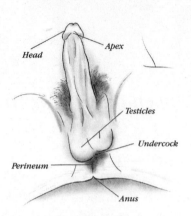

The male anatomy

e the space is created, the man being stroked removes his clothes from the waist down. This step can be confronting for a man, especially if he is not hard at the time. Men have been taught that their penises should always be erect during a sexual encounter; if not, there may be something wrong. But just as a woman is not always turned on and "ready" when the OM begins, so a man will most likely be in his resting state when he first removes his pants.

Even once the OM begins, an erection is optional. While we have become accustomed to the notion that a hard penis is *required* for a successful sexual encounter, such is not the case with OM. It is possible to stroke a man's cock even when it is soft—it simply asks more of your attention and gentleness since he may be more sensitive than you've seen him before. But the process itself is the same, whether he is hard or not. Once this truth sinks in—OM does not require him to perform in any way—the sensation can be one of great freedom and turn-on.

There are two positions that work well for male stroking.

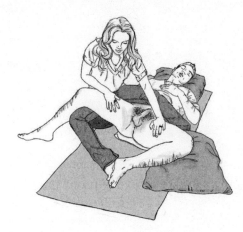

Preparing to stroke, from the traditional OM position

The first is similar to the traditional OM posture, with the stroker sitting to the right of the receiver (see the figure above).

The second posture finds the woman seated between the stroker's legs, with one of her legs over each of his thighs. This position gives a slight advantage in that it allows her to reach the cock from the front, giving her the most complete access available to his full genital region (see the figure on the next page).

Whichever position you choose, begin by placing the towel in the center of the pillows and having him lie down so it is underneath his buttocks. Help him butterfly his legs open, supporting each of his knees with a pillow or your leg. Make sure he knows that you will be taking care of everything from here on out; he doesn't need to worry about anything except relaxing. Once he is settled, take your seat beside him or between his legs. You may find it more comfortable to sit on one or more pillows; feel free to adjust as suits you best. Set the timer for fifteen minutes.

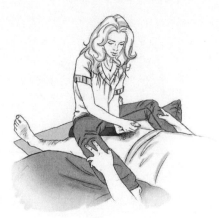

Stroking him from the alternate position, between his legs

Begin the OM with noticing. Place all your attention on his cock. Paint him a verbal portrait, focusing on color, texture, and relative location. Be objective; state just the facts. Tell him what it reminds you of, how the color moves from light to dark to light again—whatever you see. Once you have said everything that comes to mind, begin to stroke.

How to Stroke a Man

1. Place lube on your hands, gently rubbing them together to warm the lube. Let your partner know you are about to make contact.
2. Place your right hand underneath his scrotum so that his balls are lying gently in your hand. This will help him feel grounded throughout the OM.
3. Wrap your left hand around his cock so that your palm makes contact with the back side of the shaft and your thumb and fingers meet in front. (If you are

230

stroking a man who is uncircumcised, gently pull his foreskin down with your right hand, holding it there while you wrap your left hand around him.) Once your hand is in position, stroke once upward from the base of his cock to the tip, spreading lube over his shaft as you go (see figure below).

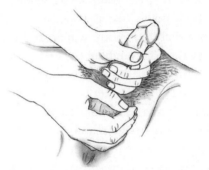

The hand position for male stroking

4. At the top of his shaft, begin to stroke slowly and lightly, focusing on an inch-long area just below the head of the penis (see figure below).

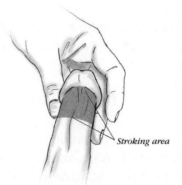

Stroking area

The most sensitive stroking area

5. Use much lighter pressure than you would normally use for a hand job, especially if his penis is not erect. Try different strokes. Firmer strokes will feel more earthy, more meaty. Lighter strokes will feel more spacious. You may rotate your hand as you stroke up and down for additional sensation if that feels good to you. Notice the melody that your stroke creates between base and high notes. See if you can sense an underlying rhythm that your body wants, and continue to stroke that rhythm. Throughout the OM, remember to tell him everything you are doing before you do it. This allows him to relax more deeply. Tell him that you are going to take a firmer grasp, or that you are going to shift the stroke. If you are the man being stroked, don't forget to ask for what you want. More or less pressure, a faster or slower stroke—whatever would feel good.

6. Both partners pay attention to the point of contact between her hand and his penis. When your minds wander, return to the sensation of her hand and his penis.

7. The man may or may not climax before the fifteen minutes is up. If he does, ask him if he would like to continue with the rest of the OM, or if he would rather go straight to the grounding step.

After the OM

Once the OM is complete, ground him by applying pressure to the shaft of his cock. You may press it against his belly or simply wrap both hands around it. You may also apply pressure to the undercock, where his shaft continues underneath the skin, below his balls. Be firm but gentle, and continue applying pressure until you feel a sort of exhale in your body and his. Then, gently pull the towel out from underneath him and use it to carefully wipe all the lube off his body. Men are especially unaccustomed to being wet down there, so make sure you are careful and thorough.

The final step is for each of you to share a frame with your partner: one sensational moment you remember from the OM. The communication of a sensation tends to magnify it and seal it into memory. Don't forget this step!

OM for Him Checklist

Ask for the OM—Feel what it feels like in your body while you do.

Set up the Space—Create the OMing "nest" for yourself and your partner. You'll want the space too be welcoming and comfortable, not too warm and not too cool, well-lit but not too bright. Make sure any distractions (like cell phones) are turned off and preferably left in another room. Gather together what you'll need:

- 3 or 4 pillows
- A yoga mat or heavy blanket, if practicing on the floor
- Lube
- Hand towel
- Timer set for fifteen minutes

Positioning—The man lies down in the middle of the pillows and butterflies his legs open. The stroker may sit in one of two positions: either to his right, in the standard OM position, or between his legs, with one of her legs over each of his hips. Either way, both his legs should be supported so he can relax, and she should sit on as many pillows as she needs to in order to be comfortable.

Noticing—The stroker places her attention on the receiver's genitals, taking them in visually. She will briefly describe what she sees to her partner, focusing on color, shape, and relative location.

Safeporting—The stroker tells her partner she is going to initiate contact. A simple, "I'm going to touch you now," is perfect.

Lube Stroke—The stroker gives one long "lube stroke," from the bottom of his cock to the top.

Stroking—She begins a short, feather-light stroke at the top of his shaft, making the stroke longer or shorter, heavier or lighter, depending on his feedback and how she feels in her own body.

Communication—Don't forget to share sensations, request a shift in stroke, or ask your partner for feedback. Strokers should continue safeporting their partner, letting him know what she is going to do before she shifts the stroke.

Two-Minute Warning—Stroker, let your partner know when there are two minutes left, simply by saying "two minutes."

Grounding—Once the stroker calls "time," she applies pressure to his genitals to ground him. She then uses the hand towel to remove any excess lube.

Sharing Frames—The partners each share a particularly memorable moment of sensation from the OM.

Further Resources

Slow Sex and Orgasmic Meditation

At OneTaste, we offer many different ways to deepen your understanding of Orgasmic Meditation, relationships, and desire, including:

- In-person classes and intensives in San Francisco and New York
- Private coaching (in-person and over the phone)
- Distance learning telecourses
- Online media
- ... and more!

Visit www.onetaste.us for more information. Or contact us at coaching@onetaste.us. or 800-994-0041 for a free consultation.

OMing Supplies

Stroking Cushions

Many strokers find that sitting on a firm cushion helps make the OMing position more comfortable. I suggest a "zafu," a round meditation cushion filled with buckwheat hulls. You can purchase zafus from many online retailers, including:

www.dharmacrafts.com
www.ziji.com
www.zafustore.com

Personal Lubricants

OneStroke—A few years back OneTaste found an all-natural lube we loved and adapted the recipe. It is a blend of olive oil, beeswax, shea butter, and grapeseed oil and is just the right consistency for OM. (It is not, however, compatible with latex condoms.) For more information and to purchase, visit www.onetaste.us.

Sliquid Organics Brand—www.sliquidorganics.com

K-Y Brand—www.drugstore.com

Organic coconut oil—www.amazon.com

The OneTaste Signature OM Kit

Everything You Need to Set Up Your Nest

The *OneTaste Signature OM Kit* contains everything you need to get started with your home practice of Orgasmic Meditation. The kit includes:

- One 100% organic cotton blanket
- One stroking cushion
- Two soft linen-covered pillows, for her legs and head
- One 2-ounce jar of handcrafted, all-natural OneStroke Lube
- Three 100% cotton hand towels

Visit www.onetaste.us for more information or to purchase.

Meditation and Mindfulness Resources

Books

Wherever You Go, There You Are by Jon Kabat-Zinn
The Wisdom of No Escape by Pema Chödrön
Seeking the Heart of Wisdom by Jack Kornfield and Joseph
  Goldstein

Guided Meditation on Audio

Mindfulness for Beginners by Jon Kabat-Zinn
How to Meditate with Pema Chödrön by Pema Chödrön
*Guided Meditation: Six Practices to Cultivate Love, Aware-
  ness, and Wisdom* by Jack Kornfield

Retreat Centers

Spirit Rock, www.spiritrock.org
Omega Institute, www.eomega.org
Shambhala International, www.shambhala.org

Acknowledgments

I don't know if you can imagine what it would be like to found a retreat center dedicated to a little-known sexuality practice, joyfully toil away for ten years in relative obscurity, and then overnight—to have people sit up and take notice. It's surreal and a bit daunting. But mostly it inspires a sense of gratitude. This practice, which I love with all my heart, is enjoying its moment in the sun.

It was Patricia Leigh Brown at the *New York Times* who saw something in OM, and in me, that was worth bringing to the world. I had been warned to be careful around reporters, but anyone who would say that has never met Patti. She is fierce and she is fair, and she gets inside to find the truth with heart. I could ask no more of any person.

When I stumbled into my agent David McCormick's office for the first time, I felt like I had fallen through a trapdoor into a sanctuary of calm sanity. What I was feeling was David himself. Suddenly I felt safe; I had a home.

Jamie Raab, Diana Baroni, and Natalie Kaire at Grand Central Publishing saw exactly what I was trying to do. At our very first meeting, I realized that I didn't have to translate for them. To land with a publisher that gets you is a gift beyond words.

Kelly Notaras has the funniest story of anyone who

has ever crossed my path. She happened on the center, not knowing what it was. A few weeks later she read the *Times* article. A few weeks after that, one of David's colleagues called her to see if she could help with the book. She signed on, and then she gave her heart to it. For this person willing to go so far beyond, I am still amazed and deeply grateful.

I cannot forget the wily bunch of orgasmic pioneers who preceded me. First and foremost, there is Ray Vetterlein, who coaxed and vexed, teased and loved my orgasm right out of me. There is Ken Blackman, who stroked me quite literally for *years* before we ever saw a little sprout come up through the cement. I am grateful to the women, especially Laura, who helped me translate this odd experience I was having called "getting turned on." To Vic, who helped me see, in the two times I met him, that I was better-suited to the orgasmic path than to the Zen center (a surprise only to me). And to the folks at the WC, who brushed and stroked my feral kitty orgasm until it was pretty and shiny.

To my myriad teachers, sisters, and guides: Lisa, Kristina, Aaron, Judy, Dean Barnlund, and Janice and Phillip Moffitt, each of whom has reconfigured my heart and mind, helping me find inspiration in the most unlikely places. And to everyone at Singularity University, for your boundless vision. I am inspired.

To Patrina, who taught me to remember to remember.

To Rob, for being willing go into every passionate no-really-*this*-one-is-it exploration with me.

To my muses, Alisha, Christina, Rachael, Rachel, and Yia. You are my daily dose of inspiration.

To the OneTaste community, past and present, who really made this possible. Your work, your passion, your belief

Acknowledgments

(despite all evidence to the contrary) is the ground on which this work rests. My sincere gratitude for all you have done, taught me, and grown this orgasm into. A special thanks to Chris and Gregg for their insight on the man stuff.

To Justine, because when U Pandita anointed us spirit friends, the word "friend" took on a whole new meaning.

Especially, and in so many ways, to my mom. With over three and a half billion women in the world, I would still choose you.

And finally, to Reese, who—after my rabbi warned me that there were likely six men in the world who could handle me, five of whom were married—is the one.

ABOUT NICOLE DAEDONE

NICOLE DAEDONE is the founder of OneTaste, a community of teachers and practitioners committed to developing innovative approaches to relationship, leadership, and healing through sexuality. The practice at the heart of her work, Orgasmic Meditation, uniquely combines the oral tradition of extended orgasm with her own interest in Zen Buddhism, mystical Judaism, and semantics.

Nicole has appeared on *Nightline*; her work has been featured in the *New York Times*, the *New York Post*, and the *San Francisco Chronicle*, among others; and her writing has appeared in *Tricycle* magazine. Still active at the San Francisco center, Nicole writes, teaches, and lectures on the relationship between language and spirituality, body and mind, and self and community.

Raised in Los Gatos, California, Nicole now lives in San Francisco with her partner, Reese Jones.

To find out more about Slow Sex and Orgasmic Meditation, visit nicoledaedone.com and onetaste.us.